*Interesting
Cases in*
Hypertension
Useful Lessons on Management

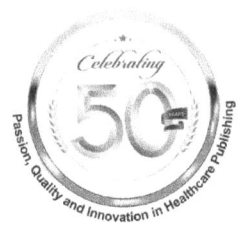

Interesting Cases in Hypertension
Useful Lessons on Management

Chief Editor

Gurpreet S Wander MD DM
Professor and Head
Department of Cardiology
Hero DMC Heart Institute
Dayanand Medical College and Hospital
Ludhiana, Punjab, India

Editors

Siddharth N Shah

YP Munjal

M Chenniappan

Falguni S Parikh

Narinder Pal Singh

Anupam Prakash

Nihar P Mehta

Vitull Gupta

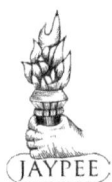

JAYPEE BROTHERS MEDICAL PUBLISHERS
The Health Sciences Publisher
New Delhi | London

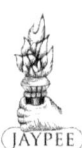 **Jaypee Brothers Medical Publishers (P) Ltd**

Headquarters
Jaypee Brothers Medical Publishers (P) Ltd
4838/24, Ansari Road, Daryaganj
New Delhi 110 002, India
Phone: +91-11-43574357
Fax: +91-11-43574314
Email: jaypee@jaypeebrothers.com

Overseas Offices
J.P. Medical Ltd
83 Victoria Street, London
SW1H 0HW (UK)
Phone: +44 20 3170 8910
Fax: +44 (0)20 3008 6180
Email: info@jpmedpub.com

Website: www.jaypeebrothers.com
Website: www.jaypeedigital.com

© 2020, Jaypee Brothers Medical Publishers

The views and opinions expressed in this book are solely those of the original contributor(s)/author(s) and do not necessarily represent those of editor(s) of the book.

All rights reserved. No part of this publication may be reproduced, stored or transmitted in any form or by any means, electronic, mechanical, photocopying, recording or otherwise, without the prior permission in writing of the publishers.

All brand names and product names used in this book are trade names, service marks, trademarks or registered trademarks of their respective owners. The publisher is not associated with any product or vendor mentioned in this book.

Medical knowledge and practice change constantly. This book is designed to provide accurate, authoritative information about the subject matter in question. However, readers are advised to check the most current information available on procedures included and check information from the manufacturer of each product to be administered, to verify the recommended dose, formula, method and duration of administration, adverse effects and contraindications. It is the responsibility of the practitioner to take all appropriate safety precautions. Neither the publisher nor the author(s)/editor(s) assume any liability for any injury and/or damage to persons or property arising from or related to use of material in this book.

This book is sold on the understanding that the publisher is not engaged in providing professional medical services. If such advice or services are required, the services of a competent medical professional should be sought.

Every effort has been made where necessary to contact holders of copyright to obtain permission to reproduce copyright material. If any have been inadvertently overlooked, the publisher will be pleased to make the necessary arrangements at the first opportunity. The **CD/DVD-ROM** (if any) provided in the sealed envelope with this book is complimentary and free of cost. **Not meant for sale.**

Inquiries for bulk sales may be solicited at: jaypee@jaypeebrothers.com

Interesting Cases in Hypertension: Useful Lessons on Management / Gurpreet S Wander

First Edition: **2020**

ISBN: 978-93-89587-59-3

Contributors

Chief Editor

Gurpreet S Wander MD DM
Professor and Head
Department of Cardiology
Hero DMC Heart Institute
Dayanand Medical College and Hospital
Ludhiana, Punjab, India

Editors

Siddharth N Shah MD FACP (Hon)
FRCP (Edin)
Consultant
Bhatia, SL Raheja, Saifee, and
Sir HN Reliance Hospitals
Mumbai, Maharashtra, India

M Chenniappan MD DM
Consultant Cardiologist
Ramakrishna Medical Centre
Tiruchirappalli, Tamil Nadu, India

Narinder Pal Singh MD MBA FRCP FACP
FISN FICP
Senior Director
Department of Internal Medicine
Max Super Speciality Hospital
Ghaziabad, Uttar Pradesh, India

Nihar P Mehta MD DNB (Medicine)
DNB (Cardiology) FRCP (London)
Consultant Cardiologist
Jaslok Hospital, Breach Candy Hospital
Sir HN Reliance and Bhatia Hospital
Mumbai, Maharashtra, India

YP Munjal MD (Medicine)
Medical Director and
Honorary Senior Consultant
Diabetes and Life Style Disease Center
Banarsidas Chandiwala Institute of
Medical Sciences
New Delhi, India

Falguni S Parikh MD DNB FICP MNAMS
Consultant
Department of Internal Medicine
Kokilaben Dhirubhai Ambani Hospital
Mumbai, Maharashtra, India

Anupam Prakash MD PGCC (Hosp Mgt)
PDCC (Dialysis Med) MAMS FICP FACP FIACM
Professor
Department of Medicine
Lady Hardinge Medical College
New Delhi, India

Vitull Gupta MD
Consultant
Department of Medicine
Kishori Ram Hospital and Diabetes
Care Centre
Bathinda, Punjab, India

Preface

We are happy to present this book which discusses some practical aspects in the management of Hypertension. We have presented case scenarios followed by some questions which the reader can answer for self. This is followed by a discussion on the topic. The answers to the questions are available in the discussion that follows. The contributing authors have all put up interesting cases with some lessons in management of your patients with hypertension. The editors are all experts in their fields with vast experience in management of these patients. Each section has been developed by an expert of the field. I have written the section on hypertension and cardiac effects.

Hypertension is the commonest non-communicable disease and has a prevalence of 28% in our country. It causes multiple target organ damage which changes the approach to management of a given case. The "Indian Guidelines on Management of Hypertension IGH- IV" were released in 2019 and should be used as a reference for management of patients. These are available on the JAPI website and can be read through the link https://japi.org/october_2019_spl/contents.html.

It is important to use the Indian guidelines since these are adapted to our population and are based on lot of data from our own country. There have been some changes in the approach to management of hypertension. The recent ACC/AHA guidelines were released in 2017 and the definition of hypertension was changed to >130/80. The subsequent ESC/ESH guidelines of 2018 and also the Indian guidelines have retained a value of >140/90 for definition of hypertension. There are many such subtle differences in approach of management which depend on the social, economic, cultural, dietary and healthcare delivery system of different countries. In this sense this book will be useful since it incorporates the experience and concepts of some experts who have managed patients with hypertension for a lifetime. It is not intended to be a textbook on hypertension. It only is a practical, useful and easy reading for guidance of clinicians regarding management of individual patients.

I have no words to express my gratitude to Mr Jitendar P Vij, Group Chairman of Jaypee Brothers Medical Publishers (P) Ltd who has taken personal interest in bringing out this book. But for his interest and guidance it would not have been possible to bring out this book. Each of the editors have contributed interesting cases, some questions and meaningful discussions. I am thankful to the staff of Jaypee Publishers specially Dr Richa, Dr Nidhi, and Himani Pandey who have made useful corrections in some of the errors that we missed as an oversight. Muskan Sharma, my secretary worked very hard to knit the whole assembly together so as to present it in the form of this beautiful book.

The ultimate aim of any academic exercise is to benefit our patients. We all will be very satisfied in case it helps to manage your patients in a better form and with evidence based.

Gurpreet S Wander

Contents

SECTION 1: HYPERTENSION AND CONCOMITANT RISK FACTORS
Siddharth N Shah

CASE 1: Hypertension and Diabetes	1
CASE 2: Hypertension and Dyslipidemia	4
CASE 3: Hypertension in Hyperuricemia	9
CASE 4: Hypertension and Obesity	14
CASE 5: Hypertension in Smokers	18

SECTION 2: HYPERTENSION – TYPES
YP Munjal

CASE 1: Resistant Hypertension	25
CASE 2: Isolated Systolic Hypertension	30
CASE 3: Downregulation of Antihypertensive Treatment	34
CASE 4: Poor Compliance in a Hypertensive	37
CASE 5: Hypertension and Wide Pulse Pressure	41

SECTION 3: INTERESTING ECGs IN HYPERTENSION
M Chenniappan

CASE 1: Left Ventricular Hypertrophy	47
CASE 2: Left Bundle Branch Block in Hypertension	50
CASE 3: Ventricular Premature Depolarizations in Hypertension	52
CASE 4: Beyond Left Ventricular Hypertrophy	53
CASE 5: The T Wave in Hypertension	55

SECTION 4: ISSUES IN DIAGNOSIS
Nihar P Mehta

CASE 1: Role of Home Blood Pressure Monitoring in Patients with Hypertension — 57

CASE 2: Role of Ambulatory Blood Pressure Monitoring in Patients with Hypertension — 61

Masked Hypertension 61
White Coat Hypertension 61
Pseudo Hypertension 62
Resistant Hypertension 62
Labile Hypertension 62

SECTION 5: HYPERTENSION IN PREGNANCY
Falguni S Parikh

CASE 1: Pregnancy in Aortoarteritis — 65
CASE 2: Pre-eclampsia — 68
CASE 3: Chronic Hypertension in Pregnancy — 71
CASE 4: Eclampsia — 74
CASE 5: Hypertension in Postpartum Period — 76

SECTION 6: HYPERTENSION AND RENAL DISORDERS
Narinder Pal Singh

CASE 1: Hypertension in Patient with Glomerular Filtration Rate <15 — 80
CASE 2: Hypertension in Patient with Glomerular Filtration Rate 30–60 — 83
CASE 3: Hypertension in Patient with Microalbuminuria — 85
CASE 4: Nephritic Illness with Hypertension — 90
CASE 5: Chronic Kidney Disease Patient on Dialysis with Hypertension — 94

SECTION 7: CEREBROVASCULAR ASSOCIATIONS
Vitull Gupta

CASE 1: Hypertension in Acute Hemorrhagic Stroke — 98
CASE 2: Hypertension in Acute Ischemic Stroke — 107
CASE 3: Hypertension with Subarachnoid Hemorrhage — 113
CASE 4: Hypertensive Encephalopathy — 125
CASE 5: Post Stroke Patient with Hypertension — 133

SECTION 8: SECONDARY HYPERTENSION CASES
Anupam Prakash

CASE 1: Pheochromocytoma — 138
CASE 2: Conn Syndrome — 141
CASE 3: Thyrotoxicosis with Hypertension — 144
CASE 4: Hypothyroidism with Hypertension — 147
CASE 5: Cushing's with Hypertension — 149

SECTION 9: CARDIAC EFFECTS
Gurpreet S Wander

CASE 1: Hypertension and Heart Failure with a Preserved Ejection Fraction — 152
CASE 2: Hypertension and Coronary Artery Disease — 157
CASE 3: Hypertension and Heart Failure — 162
CASE 4: Hypertension and Acute Myocardial Infarction — 167
CASE 5: Hypertension and Atrial Fibrillation — 172

What is New in Indian Guidelines on Hypertension-IV? — 177

Index — 179

SECTION 1
Hypertension and Concomitant Risk Factors

Siddharth N Shah

CASE 1: Hypertension and Diabetes

A 65-year-old hypertensive female came to OPD with complaint of headache. She is a known diabetic since 10 years on insulin therapy. Her medications included tablet amlodipine 5 mg twice a day and tablet hydrochlorothiazide 12.5 mg once daily.

On examination, her heart rate was 96 beats/min and blood pressure was 166/100 mm Hg. Her respiratory rate was 14 breaths/min. The cardiovascular (CV) examination was essentially normal with no S_3 or S_4. Her urine routine showed 2+ proteinuria. An electrocardiogram did not demonstrate ischemic changes and was within normal limits.

Baseline echocardiography showed normal left ventricular (LV) systolic and diastolic function and no regional wall motion abnormalities.

Q1. Which of the following drugs should be first line for hypertension control?
   a. Angiotensin-converting enzyme (ACE) inhibitor
   b. Mineralocorticoid receptor antagonist
   c. Beta-blockers
   d. Calcium channel blocker

Q2. Target systolic blood pressure in diabetics as per JNC 8 and Indian Hypertension Guidelines-III is:
   a. <130 mm Hg
   b. <120 mm Hg
   c. <140 mm Hg
   d. <150 mm Hg

Q3. Which of the following statements is correct?
   a. Angiotensin receptor blockers (ARBs) are preferred over ACE inhibitors in diabetics
   b. Hypertension is less common in diabetics as compared to nondiabetics
   c. Most diabetic hypertensive patients need two or more antihypertensive drugs for target control
   d. None of the above

Q4. Which combination regimen is found to be most superior in diabetics?
   a. ACE inhibitor and calcium channel blocker
   b. ACE inhibitor and thiazide diuretic
   c. Beta-blocker and thiazide diuretic
   d. ACE inhibitor and beta-blocker

Q5. Which of the following statements is incorrect?
   a. Beta-blockers are relatively contraindicated in diabetic patients
   b. Chlorthalidone is associated with increased incidence of new onset diabetes
   c. Thiazides not effective in chronic kidney disease (CKD) stage 3 or more patients (i.e., GFR <60 mL/min/1.73 m^2)
   d. None of the above

Ans. 1-a, 2-b, 3-c, 4-a, 5-a

DISCUSSION

Nearly 70% of the patients with diabetes are affected by hypertension, which is twice the rate that is noticed in nondiabetic individuals. There exists a steep-graded association between adverse cardiovascular (CV) outcomes and blood pressure. Numerous classes of antihypertensive medications reduce diabetic cardiovascular disease (CVD) risk, and given the potent benefits for both macrovascular and microvascular disease complications, blood pressure management is of principal importance in this high-risk population.

For explaining the association that exists between diabetes mellitus and hypertension, many pathogenic mechanisms have been proposed. These are believed to be mediated via the role of the adrenergic system in both, diabetes mellitus as well as hypertension. These mechanisms comprise of the incretin-mediated control of the renin–angiotensin–aldosterone system (RAAS). Additionally, in both of these disorders, the calcium–calmodulin pathway has been studied extensively. Changes in the calcium–calmodulin system lead to increased intracellular calcium levels; this has been shown to inhibit transcription of the insulin gene in pancreatic beta-cells. Such alterations result in extracellular fluid expansion, increase in arterial stiffness, and development of diabetic nephropathy. Interestingly, the studies demonstrate that patients with uncontrolled BP in spite of antihypertensive therapy have been shown to be at a higher risk for developing diabetes mellitus.

Treatment of Hypertension in Diabetics

Special attention should be given to diabetic patients with hypertension. The two commonly coexist and multiply the CV risks of each alone. Evidence from several trials has now documented the protection provided by intensive control of hypertension, in concert with management of the diabetes and the dyslipidemia that commonly accompanies the two.

Current Guidelines
Indian Hypertension Guidelines-IV (2019) recommend threshold for treatment and goal BP of >140/80 mm Hg.

Antihypertensive Therapy

Five classes of medications have substantial evidence basis for CVD efficacy in the setting of diabetes, including ACE inhibitors, calcium channel blockers, beta-blockers, thiazide diuretics, and angiotensin II receptor blockers (ARBs).

Angiotensin-converting Enzyme Inhibitors

The recommendation for ACE inhibitors as first-line hypertension therapy in the setting of diabetes is supported by data from randomized trials of patients with and without hypertension. For example, in the HOPE (Heart Outcomes Prevention Evaluation) study, which compared ramipril versus placebo among patients at increased risk for CVD, ramipril was superior to placebo in the diabetes subset of 3,577 HOPE patients. Especially in patients with nephropathy and proteinuria, ACE inhibitors are most preferred drugs.

Angiotensin II Receptor Blockers

Cardiovascular outcomes data for ARBs are much less robust than for ACE inhibitors and are particularly lacking for patients with diabetes. The TRANSCEND (Telmisartan Randomized AssessmeNt Study in ACE iNtolerant subjects with cardiovascular Disease) trial, telmisartan did not achieve statistical superiority over placebo in reducing the primary composite. ARBs should be considered second-line therapy, and their use reserved for those patients who cannot tolerate ACE inhibitors because of cough, angioedema, or rash.

Beta-blockers

Earlier beta-blockers were considered relatively contraindicated in the setting of diabetes because of concerns about masking hypoglycemia symptoms and adverse effects on glucose and lipid metabolism. The concerns have been mitigated with research supporting the benefit of beta-blockers for patients with diabetes in the chronic ambulatory setting and in the post-ACS population. The utility of beta-blockers in the treatment of patients with diabetes has most recently been supported by a meta-analysis of randomized clinical trials.

Thiazide Diuretics

Concerns about the adverse glycometabolic effects of the thiazide diuretic class of medications have resulted in some degree of hesitancy to use these medications in diabetics. However, randomized trials of thiazide diuretics that included substantial numbers of patients with diabetes have consistently demonstrated CVD benefits despite their adverse metabolic effects. In a subanalysis of the ALLHAT (Antihypertensive and Lipid-Lowering Treatment to Prevent Heart Attack Trial), the CVD effects of chlorthalidone compared with both lisinopril and amlodipine were similar in patients with diabetes or impaired fasting glucose, despite modest but statistically significant increases in incident diabetes associated with chlorthalidone.

Calcium Channel Blockers

Dihydropyridine calcium channel blockers are well tolerated and effective at lowering blood pressure in diabetics. Analyses of diabetes subsets of randomized clinical trials have suggested CVD clinical benefits of a magnitude similar to or greater than those observed in the nondiabetic cohorts, including evaluations of nitrendipine, nisoldipine, and amlodipine. In randomized trials directly comparing the efficacy of calcium channel blockers versus ACE inhibitors, superior outcomes were observed with ACE inhibitors.

Combination Therapy

Number of studies have also demonstrated the benefits of combination therapy in patients with diabetes. In the ACCOMPLISH (Avoiding Cardiovascular Events through Combination Therapy in Patients Living with Systolic Hypertension) trial, all patients were treated with benazepril, with randomization to add-on amlodipine versus add-on hydrochlorothiazide, treatment with benazepril–amlodipine versus benazepril–hydrochlorothiazide was associated with a 21% reduction in CVD outcomes.

KEY POINTS

- Five classes of medications have substantial evidence basis for CVD efficacy in the setting of diabetes including ACE inhibitors, calcium channel blockers, beta-blockers, thiazide diuretics, and ARBs. Aggressive blood pressure control for patients with diabetes to achieve optimal CVD risk mitigation is required. Most patients require a combination of multiple blood pressure medications to achieve strict control.

SUGGESTED READING

1. Cryer MJ, Horani T, DiPette DJ. Diabetes and hypertension. A comparative review of current guidelines. J Clin Hypertens (Greenwich). 2016;18(2):95-100.
2. Jamerson K, Weber MA, Bakris GL, et al. Benazepril plus amlodipine or hydrochlorothiazide for hypertension in high-risk patients. N Engl J Med. 2008;359(23):2417-28.
3. Turnbull F, Neal B, Algert C, et al. Effects of different blood pressure-lowering regimens on major cardiovascular events in individuals with and without diabetes mellitus: Results of prospectively designed overviews of randomized trials. Arch Intern Med. 2005;165(12):1410-9.

CASE 2: Hypertension and Dyslipidemia

A 52-year-old male came to OPD with routine follow-up of BP. He is hypertensive for last 10 years on tablets amlodipine and losartan. There is no history of angina or any renal disease. He had a BMI of 29 kg/m^2.

On evaluation, his BP was 160/94 mm Hg, ECG showed left ventricular hypertrophy (LVH), and echocardiography showed grade I diastolic dysfunction (DD). Serum creatinine was 0.9, routine urine examination was normal, and lipid profile showed total cholesterol: 243 mg/dL, LDL: 140 mg/dL, HDL: 34 mg/dL, and triglyceride: 194 mg/dL.

Q1. Which of the following measures are helpful in a patient with metabolic syndrome?
   a. Angiotensin II receptor blockers
   b. Statin
   c. Increased physical activity
   d. All of the above

Q2. All of the following are the components of metabolic syndrome except:
   a. Triglyceride >150 mg/dL
   b. LDL-C >200 mg/dL
   c. Central obesity
   d. FBS >100 mg/dL

Q3. Therapeutic lifestyle changes in case of increased LDL include:
   a. Weight reduction
   b. Increased physical activity
   c. Saturated fat <7% of calories, increased soluble fibers 10–25 g/day
   d. All of the above

Ans. 1-d, 2-b, 3-d

DISCUSSION

Worldwide, there is an increase in the burden of cardiovascular disease (CVD). In developing countries, such as India, one of the major concerns is increase in the burden of CVD. It is proven that the two major contributing risk factors for CVD are hypertension and dyslipidemia. The prevalence of the coexistence of hypertension and dyslipidemia, as demonstrated by several epidemiological studies, is found to be in the range of 15–31%. It has been demonstrated that when two risk factors coexist, they have more than an additive adverse effect on the vascular endothelium; this leads to increased atherosclerosis, further resulting in CVD. "Lipitension" is the term which stands for "coexistence and interplay of dyslipidemia and hypertension".

According to the NCEP (National Cholesterol Education Program) Guidelines (Adult Treatment Panel III), they comprise the vital components of the metabolic syndrome (MS).[1]

It has been invariably demonstrated by studies that there is frequent co-existence of hypertension and hypercholesterolemia, which leads to dyslipidemic hypertension (DH).[2,3] The risk of CVD that is associated with concomitant hypertension and dyslipidemia is shown to be more multiplicative as compared to the sum of the individual risk factors.[4,5]

The Interplay—Lipitension

Dyslipidemia is one the strong predictors of CVD. It results in the endothelial damage as well as loss of physiological vasomotor activity.[6,7] There is a continuous and consistent relationship of blood pressure with the risk of cardiovascular (CV) events. The chances of CVD increase as per the increase in the BP. The risk for hypertension is multiplied by the presence of each added risk factor. There is, however, limited evidence of the effect of high BP on lipid levels.

In a large epidemiological study, MRFIT (Multiple Risk Factor Intervention Trial), this interplay of lipitension was noted. Findings of this study emphasized that there was a multiplicative adverse impact of even mild-to-moderate levels of both hypertension and dyslipidemia on the risk for coronary heart disease (CHD). The risk was comparable or more because of a severe increase in either one of the risk factors. Moreover, it was also reported by the findings of the Framingham Study that moderate elevation in BP as well as cholesterol had a comparable 10-year risk of CHD, in comparison to those with highly increased systolic BP or LDL cholesterol alone.[8]

Lipitension and Atherosclerosis

Atherogenesis is promoted by the renin–angiotensin–aldosterone system (RAAS). Angiotensin II is considered to be a main villain of the RAAS pathway. Atherogenesis is promoted via stimulation of the angiotensin type 1 receptor (AT1) which enhances uptake of lipid in cells, vasoconstriction as well as free radical production, for promoting both hypertension and atherosclerosis.[9]

Endothelium is damaged by hypertension due to the altered shear stress and oxidative stress. This leads to increase in endothelial cell synthesis of collagen and fibronectin and increase in permeability to lipoproteins and decrease in nitric oxide-dependent vascular relaxation.[10,11] There is also an association of hypertension with an upregulation of lipid oxidation enzymes.[12] A major cause of endothelial dysfunction is LDL, specifically oxidized LDL.[13] Therefore, due to its effects on the level of the endothelium, lipitension contributes to atherosclerosis as well as the resultant vascular risk.

Effect of Lipid-lowering Therapy on Blood Pressure

Some evidence exists which demonstrate that treating dyslipidemia has beneficial effects on BP. Borghi et al.[14,15] reported that patients who receive concomitant antihypertensive and statin therapy showed decrease in BP; it was suggested that using statins along with antihypertensive drugs can improve control of BP in patients who have uncontrolled hypertension and elevated levels of serum cholesterol.

The pathophysiological basis behind the apparent advantageous impact of statin therapy on BP may be because of the positive effects of statins on endothelial or vascular smooth muscle cell functions or both. BP can also be influenced by hypercholesterolemia by potentiating the impact on the endothelium of the vasoconstrictors angiotensin II and endothelin-1.[16-18] Therefore, a decrease in production of nitric oxide, along with an increased vasoconstrictor response, will result in elevated BP in patients who have dyslipidemia.

Effect of Blood Pressure Lowering Therapy on Lipid Levels

There is a certain impact of blood pressure lowering drugs on the lipid levels. Amongst all of the antihypertensive drugs, changes in the lipid parameters have been showed by beta-blockers and thiazide diuretics. There is little impact of selective blockers (beta-1) and newer beta-blockers on the levels of total cholesterol. At higher doses, the effect of thiazide diuretics on cholesterol parameters becomes apparent.

Considering the effect on plasma lipid alpha-blockers, the calcium channel blocker or the RAAS blocker may be the preferred initial therapy in patients with underlying hyperlipidemia.

Lipitension and Coronary Artery Disease

In coronary artery disease (CAD) patients, lipitension, as a combination, is one of the important risk factors for the progression of atherosclerosis. Adnan et al. in their study evaluated the effect of the optimal control of LDL-C as well as systolic BP on the progression of atheroma in the coronary arteries by using the intravascular ultrasound (IVUS). It was concluded that the patients who had very low LDL-C (<70 mg/dL) and normal systolic BP (SBP) (≤120 mm Hg) showed the least progression of percentage atheroma ($p < 0.001$) as well as more frequent plaque regression ($p < 0.01$). It is suggested by findings of this study that there is a need for the intensive control of lipitension as a part of global risk factors among patients who have CAD.[19]

Conversely, it has been demonstrated by some of the trials, such as the BCAP (Beta-Blocker Cholesterol-Lowering Asymptomatic Plaque) study and ELVA, that there are beneficial effects of beta-blocker therapy on decreasing early progression of atherosclerosis and thickening of intima-media thickness (IMT), among asymptomatic patients having carotid plaque, in addition to decrease of BP. This also leads to a reduction in CVD mortality.[20,21]

■ MANAGEMENT

One of the major causes of endothelial dysfunction is LDL. Microalbuminuria is identified in hypertensive patients. It is also associated with lipid abnormalities such as increased LDL and TGL levels, reduced HDL levels, and increased LP(a) levels. Prevention of CVD is focused on treatment of hypertension with the reducing LDL (<100 mg%), enhancing HDL (>40 mg in males), and reducing TGL (<150 mg%). ACE inhibitors, ARBs, aldosterone antagonists, and nebivolol improve endothelial function and reduce BP. Statin treatment happens to be as a first line drug therapy in the management of dyslipidemia. Fibrates are generally reserved for hypertriglyceridemia. Bile sequestrants, nicotinic acid, and drugs like ezetimibe locally acting at the intestine level are also used for dyslipidemia. Single pill combinations like atorvastatin with RASS blocker/amlodipine may be considered the coexisting hypertension and dyslipidemia.

KEY POINTS

- Well-known risk factors for CVD include dyslipidemia and hypertension. It has been proved that the coexistence of both these conditions has adverse outcomes. Worldwide, there is variation in prevalence of coexistence. Interaction takes place at the vascular endothelial level between these two risk factors. This leads to increase in oxidative stress, endothelial dysfunction as well as progression of atherosclerosis. This ends up with a major CV event.
- The usual focus is more on insulin resistance as well as lipid levels, while treating the metabolic syndrome, ignoring BP. A novel approach for tackling the coexistence of hypertension and dyslipidemia is therefore required.

REFERENCES

1. Bethesda: National Heart, Lung, and Blood Institute. (2001). Third Report of the National Cholesterol Education Program (NCEP) Expert Panel. Detection, evaluation and treatment of high blood cholesterol in adults (Adult Treatment Panel III). NIH Publication No. 01-3670. [online] Available from nhlbi.nih.gov/files/docs/guidelines/atp3xsum.pdf [Last accessed December, 2019].
2. Williams RR, Hunt SC, Hopkins PN, et al. Familial dyslipidemic hypertension: Evidence from 58 Utah families for a syndrome present in approximately 12% of patients with essential hypertension. JAMA. 1988;259(24):3579-86.
3. Kannel WB. Fifty years of Framingham study contributions to understanding hypertension. J Hum Hypertens. 2000;14(2):83-90.
4. Stamler J, Wentworth D, Neaton D. Prevalence and prognostic significance of hyper-cholesterolemia in men with hypertension: Prospective data on the primary screenees of the Multiple Risk Factor Intervention Trial. Am J Med. 1986;80(2A):33-9.
5. Castelli P, Anderson K. A population at risk: Prevalence of high cholesterol levels in hypertensive patients in the Framingham Study. Am J Med. 1986; 80(2A):23-32.
6. Wong ND, Lopez V, Tang S, et al. Prevalence, treatment, and control of combined hypertension and hypercholesterolemia in adults in the USA. Am J Cardiol. 2006;98:204-8.
7. Nickenig G, Harrison G. The AT (1)-type angiotensin receptor in oxidative stress and atherogenesis: Part I: Oxidative stress and atherogenesis. Circulation. 2002;105(3):393-6.
8. Liao D, Mo J, Duan Y, et al. The joint effect of hypertension and elevated LDL-cholesterol on CHD is beyond additive. Eur Heart J. 2004;25(Suppl):S235.
9. Ross R. Atherosclerosis an inflammatory disease. N Engl J Med. 1999;340(2):115-26.
10. O'Donnell VB. Free radicals and lipid signaling in endothelial cells. Antiox Redox Signal. 2003;5:195-203.
11. Wolfrum S, Jensen KS, Liao JK. Endothelium-dependent effects of statins. Arterioscler Thromb Vasc Biol. 2003;23(5):729-36.

12. Kaplan M, Aviram M. Oxidized low density lipoprotein: atherogenic and proinflammatory characteristics during macrophage foam cell formation. An inhibitory role for nutritional antioxidants and serum paraoxonase. Clin Chem Lab Med. 1999;37(8):777-87.
13. Campese VM, Bianchi S, Bigazzi R. Association between hyperlipidemia and microalbuminuria in essential hypertension. Kidney Int. 1999;56(Suppl 71):S10-3.
14. Borghi C, Prandin G, Costa V, et al. Use of statins and blood pressure control in treated hypertensive patients with hypercholesterolemia. J Cardiovasc Pharmacol. 2000;35(4): 549-55.
15. Borghi C, Dormi A, Veronesi M, et al. Association between different lipid-lowering treatment strategies and blood pressure control in the Brisighella Heart Study. Am Heart J. 2004;148(2):285-92.
16. Cardillo C, Kilcoyne CM, Cannon RO, et al. Increased activity of endogenous endothelin in patients with hypercholesterolemia. J Am Coll Cardiol. 2000;36(5):1483-8.
17. Wierzbicki AS. Lipid lowering: Another method of reducing blood pressure? J Hum Hypertens. 2002;16(11):753-60.
18. Working Group on Management of Patients with Hypertension and High Blood Cholesterol. National education programs working group report on the management of patients with hypertension and high blood cholesterol. Ann Intern Med. 1991;114:224.
19. Hedblad B, Wikstrand J, Janzon L, et al. Low-dose metoprolol CR/XL and fluvastatin slow progression of carotid intima-media thickness: Main results from the ß-Blocker Cholesterol-Lowering Asymptomatic Plaque Study (BCAPS). Circulation. 2001;103(13):1721-6.
20. Wiklund O, Hulthe J, Wikstrand J, et al. Effect of controlled release/extended release metoprolol on carotid intima-media thickness in patients with hypercholesterolemia: A 3-Year Randomized Study. Stroke. 2002;33:572-7.
21. Hart JT. Rule of halves: Implications of increasing diagnosis and reducing dropout for future workload and prescribing costs in primary care. Br J Gen Pract. 1992;42:116-9.

CASE 3: Hypertension in Hyperuricemia

A 66-year-old hypertensive male came to OPD with complaints of severe pain in right great toe since past 15 days. His medications included tablet amlodipine 5 mg twice a day and tablet hydrochlorothiazide 12.5 mg once daily.

On examination, his heart rate was 96 beats/min and blood pressure was 160/100 mm Hg. His respiratory rate was 14 breaths/min. Patient's wrists and right MTP joints were tender, swollen, and erythematous.

Cardiovascular examination was essentially normal with no S_3 or S_4.

The electrocardiogram was within normal limits. Baseline echocardiography showed concentric left ventricular hypertrophy (LVH) with normal LV systolic and no regional wall motion abnormalities.

Q1. Which of the following drugs does not cause hyperuricemia?
   a. Thiazides and loop diuretics
   b. Statins
   c. Pyrazinamide
   d. Low-dose aspirin

Q2. Which of the following is the true regarding the development of hypertension in patients with hyperuricemia?
 a. Chronic hyperuricemia stimulates the renin–angiotensin–aldosterone system and inhibits the release of endothelial nitric oxide
 b. Increased reactive oxygen species and the decreased nitric oxide leads to renal vascular inflammation
 c. Vasoreactive hypertension evolves to a salt-sensitive hypertension
 d. All of the above

Q3. Which is not true about hypertension associated with raised serum urate levels?
 a. Increased serum uric acid level results in hypertension within 2 weeks
 b. The increases in systolic blood pressure (SBP) and diastolic blood pressure (DBP) are proportional to those of uric acid levels
 c. It can be ameliorated by uric acid lowering drugs like allopurinol
 d. None of the above

Q4. Which is not true about uric acid metabolism?
 a. Diets rich in fatty meats, seafood, and alcohol increase serum uric acid
 b. Serum uric acid levels also correlate with sweetener consumption
 c. Approximately 15% of uric acid clearance is through the gastrointestinal tract (GIT); consequently, small bowel disease can also contribute to increased serum uric acid
 d. None of the above

Q5. Which of the following statements is not true?
 a. Early hypertension is completely reversible with urate reduction, but prolonged hyperuricemia results in irreversible sodium-sensitive hypertension
 b. Obesity confers a 3-fold increased risk of hyperuricemia
 c. A rise in the serum uric acid levels by 1 mg/dL increases the SBP and DBP by 28 mm Hg and 15 mm Hg, respectively in nonobese young men
 d. None of the above

Ans. 1-b, 2-d, 3-d, 4-d, 5-d

INTRODUCTION

Several studies have proposed that there is an association between hyperuricemia and hypertension. It has been proved that levels of serum uric acid are an independent predictor for development of hypertension. Regardless of the different ethnic origins, a continuous relationship between serum uric acid and blood pressure was observed in African-Americans and Whites and in Asians including Koreans. Mazzali et al. evaluated the causal role of serum uric acid in the development of hypertension in rat models. It was observed that there was an increase in levels of serum uric acid followed by an elevation in blood pressure via a crystal-independent mechanism.

EPIDEMIOLOGY

The prevalence of gout has been increasing. As per the estimation made by the NHANES III (Third National Health and Nutrition Examination Survey), in 1994, >5 million Americans were affected by gout. Data generated NHANES (2007-2008) reported that amongst those with history of gout, 74% had hypertension while 47% of those with hyperuricemia but no history of gout, had hypertension.

PHYSIOLOGY AND METABOLISM OF URIC ACID

Due to the westernized lifestyle and environment, frequency of hyperuricemia and gout is on a rise. Though the physiological solubility of uric acid occurs at 6.4 mg/dL, the presence of uric acid-binding proteins raises this solubility up to 7.0 mg/dL prior to achieving a supersaturated state. It is due to this reason that hyperuricemia takes place when the serum uric acid levels exceeds 7.0 mg/dL, which is the point when uric acid begins to crystalize inside the human body. An enhanced level of serum uric acid accompanies the enhanced risk of disease that is related to adult lifestyle habits (i.e., lifestyle diseases), even when the level of serum uric acid is ≤7.0 mg/dL. In comparison to men, the risk of disease increases at even reduced levels of serum uric acid and needs more attention in women.

About 15% of uric acid clearance takes place via the GIT; small bowel disease can therefore also result in enhanced serum uric acid. Diets that are rich in fatty meats, seafood, and alcohol enhance the level of serum uric acid. Obesity confers a 3-fold increase in the risk of hyperuricemia. Renal clearance of uric acid can be altered by many medications, even when glomerular filtration rate is normal, consisting of loop and thiazide diuretics. These can signify an uncommon cause of hyperuricemia. Since the endpoint of the purine disposal pathway is uric acid, serum uric acid will be increased due to impairment of the efficiency of purine recycling metabolism or overwhelming the recycling pathway with cell turnover or excessive cell death. There is also a correlation between serum uric acid levels and consumption of sweetener.

ROLE OF HYPERURICEMIA IN THE DEVELOPMENT OF HYPERTENSION

Early hypertension is completely reversible with urate reduction, but prolonged hyperuricemia results in irreversible sodium-sensitive hypertension that becomes uric acid independent. The early hypertension, mediated by enhanced renal renin activity as well as decrease in circulating plasma nitrates, results in a phenotype of excessive vasoconstriction, which can be reversed by decreasing uric acid or renin–angiotensin system blockade. The later irreversible hypertension is secondary to altered intrarenal vascular architecture. Through the uric acid anion transporter-1 channel, uric acid enters the vascular smooth muscle cells, leading to activation of kinases, nuclear transcription factors, generation of cyclooxygenase-2, and the platelet-derived growth factors (PDGFs) and inflammatory proteins (monocyte chemoattractant protein-1 (MCP-1), C-reactive protein) leading to the shifted pressure natriuresis, proliferation of vascular smooth muscle cells, and sodium-sensitive hypertension (**Fig. 1**).

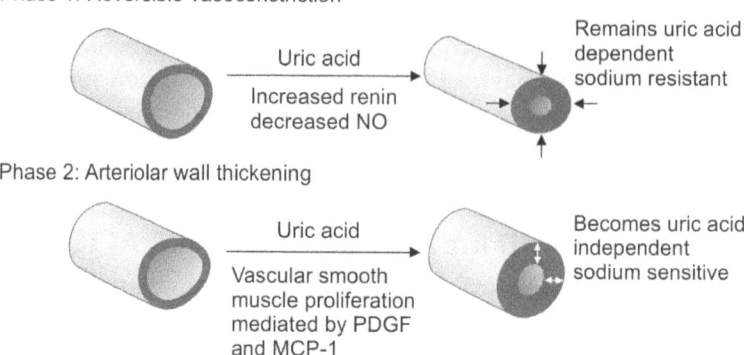

(MCP-1: monocyte chemoattractant protein-1; PDGF: platelet-derived growth factor)

Fig. 1: Role of uric acid.

The animal studies indicate that early in the disease, the renin–angiotensin system of the body is activated by the extra uric acid, leading to shrinking of key blood vessels and causing high blood pressure.

Finally, the small vessels in the kidney, however, are permanently affected, which makes the blood pressure sensitive to sodium or salt. Excess of salt causes the pressure to rise.

According to a JAMA study conducted by Feig et al., teens, who had newly diagnosed high blood pressure and increased uric acid levels in their blood, were treated with allopurinol. In this study, half of the 30 teenagers, who were newly diagnosed with high blood pressure and had higher than normal levels of uric acid in their blood, underwent treatment with allopurinol twice a day for 4 weeks. On the same schedule, the remaining 50% received a placebo (which was an inactive drug). After that, they remained without either drug for 2 weeks prior to getting the opposite treatment for another 4 weeks. With this treatment, not only the uric acid levels were reduced, but also the blood pressure was reduced in most of the teens. In 20 out of the 30 teens, blood pressure reduced to normal when receiving allopurinol. On the contrary, only 1 out of the 30 teens had normal blood pressure when they were on placebo.

■ DIURETICS, HYPERTENSION, AND HYPERURICEMIA (TABLE 1)

Hyperuricemia is caused by both thiazide and loop diuretics. The polyarticular gout characterized by tophi over the distal phalangeal joints of older persons taking diuretics has been well described. According to a prospective, population-based study from USA conducted by McAdams-DeMarco et al., the cumulative incidence of gout amongst the diuretic and nondiuretic users was 5.5% and 2.9%, respectively.

Even in the individuals without hypertension, angiotensin-converting enzyme (ACE) inhibitors, beta-blockers, diuretics, and nonlosartan angiotensin II receptor blockers (ARBs) were found to be associated with enhanced risk of gout. Hydrochlorothiazide was the most common.

TABLE 1: Multivariate relative risks of incident gout with current antihypertensive drugs in those with hypertension (n = 10,195).

Calcium channel antagonists	0.87	(0.82–0.93)
Losartan	0.78	(0.67–0.92)
Diuretics	2.35	(2.19–2.53)
Beta-blockers	1.49	(1.40–1.59)
ACE inhibitors	1.25	(1.17–1.22)
Nonlosartan ARB	1.31	(1.17–1.47)

(ACE: angiotensin-converting enzyme; ARB: angiotensin II receptor blocker)

Among the antihypertensive drugs, losartan is an exception, as it possesses mild uricosuric properties. Thus, it plays a role in treatment of patients with hypertension who have gout. The hypouricemic importance of losartan is well documented; it is believed to block the tubular organic acid transporter URAT1 resulting in enhanced excretion of urate.

Management of hyperuricemia that is induced by diuretic is based mainly on clinical experience. One of the options is to reduce the dose of thiazide instead of discontinuing it. It is because drug-related hyperuricemia is dose-related. In such cases, spironolactone may be a good add-on.

KEY POINTS

- In epidemiological studies, hypertension is found to be a common associate of hyperuricemia as well as gout. There is a complex cause and effect relationship of both hyperuricemia and hypertension with alcohol, diuretic use, obesity, and renal impairment.
- There is unconfirmed evidence that serum urate levels influence blood pressure through the renin–angiotensin system and by accelerating renovascular disease.
- Treatment of hypertension with diuretics is a common cause of hyperuricemia in individuals; it is hard to overcome with allopurinol. Patients who have increased levels of uric acid may be more quick to respond to uric acid-lowering treatment early in the course of their disease.
- Allopurinol and probenecid are not optimal options for preventive therapy because they have side effect profiles, which are inferior to conventional antihypertensive medication.
- For controlling hypertension in such patients, among the ARBs, the uricosuric effect of losartan is unique. An option is to discontinue or reduce the thiazide dose as drug-related hyperuricemia is dose-related.

SUGGESTED READING

1. Gibson TJ. Hypertension, its treatment, hyperuricaemia and gout. Curr Opin Rheumatol. 2013;25(2):217-22.
2. Feig DI. Hyperuricemia and hypertension. Adv Chronic Kidney Dis. 2012;19(6):377-85.

CASE 4: Hypertension and Obesity

A 65-year-old hypertensive female, morbidly obese with BMI of 32, came to OPD with complain of headache. Her medications included tablet amlodipine 5 mg twice a day.

On examination, her heart rate was 86 beats/min and blood pressure was 166/100 mm Hg. Her respiratory rate was 14 breaths/min. Cardiovascular (CV) examination was essentially normal with no S_3 or S_4. An electrocardiogram did not demonstrate ischemic changes and was within normal limits.

Baseline echocardiography showed normal left ventricular (LV) systolic and diastolic function and no regional wall motion abnormalities.

Q1. Which of the following factors are associated with obesity and hypertension?
   a. Renin–angiotensin stimulation with inappropriately high circulating plasma levels of aldosterone
   b. Insulin resistant state
   c. Stimulation of the sympathetic nervous system
   d. Obstructive sleep apnea syndrome
   e. All of the above

Q2. Management strategies for resistant hypertension in obese include:
   a. Mineralocorticoid antagonist
   b. Direct renin inhibitor
   c. Renal sympathetic denervation
   d. Baroreflex activation therapy
   e. All of the above

Q3. Which of the following statements is correct?
   a. Hypertension has equal incidence in obese as is in the normal subjects
   b. Hypertension occurs more commonly in obese with non-central fat depositions as compared to those with central (visceral fat distribution)
   c. Most obese hypertensive patients need two or more antihypertensive drugs for target control and are prone to resistant and refractory hypertension
   d. None of the above

Q4. Leptins stimulate hypertension by:
   a. Activation of sympathetic nervous system
   b. Direct vasoconstriction
   c. Activation of RAAS
   d. Sodium retention

Q5. Which of the following statements is incorrect in obese patients?
   a. ACE-inhibitors are first-line antihypertensives for most patients

b. Angiotensin II receptor blockers can be used in patients who do not tolerate angiotensin-converting enzyme inhibition
c. Beta-blockers are less effective in decreasing blood pressure in obese than in lean hypertensive individuals
d. Dihydropyridine calcium channel blocker related peripheral edema is more common in obese patients

Ans. 1-e, 2-e, 3-c, 4-a, 5-c

DISCUSSION

Worldwide, one of the major threats to global health is obesity as well as its associated metabolic, cardiovascular, and renal disorders. Since 1980, obesity has approximately doubled across the globe. According to the current estimates, >1.4 billion adults are overweight or obese.

Researches in different population around the globe have demonstrated that the association between body mass index (BMI) and systolic blood pressure (SBP) and diastolic blood pressure (DBP) is approximately linear. Risk estimates from the Framingham Heart Study suggest that excess weight gain is responsible for primary (essential) hypertension in 78% of men and 65% of women. It is reported by clinical studies that in primary prevention of hypertension, maintaining BMI <25 kg/m^2 is effective.

In majority of patients with hypertension, weight loss lowers BP. It has been estimated that for every 10% rise in body weight, there is an increase of 6.5 mm Hg in SBP.

For explaining the association between obesity and hypertension, many pathogenic mechanisms have been proposed. Obesity-related hypertension is usually accompanied by:
- Blood volume overload
- Stimulation of renin–angiotensin with inappropriately high circulating plasma aldosterone levels
- Insulin-resistant state
- Sympathetic nervous system stimulation
- Obstructive sleep apnea syndrome (that further complicates the obese state).

When evaluating and treating patients with obesity-related hypertension, the overall cardiovascular risk as well as secondary causes of hypertension should be taken into account, similar to approaches followed in all patients with hypertension. This is specifically compelling due to the association of obesity-related hypertension with dyslipidemia, insulin resistance, as well as type 2 diabetes mellitus (T2DM). General treatment guidelines (changes in lifestyle and diet) which are followed for the treatment of all patients with hypertension are also relevant for obesity-related hypertension.

Drug-resistant hypertension is defined as BP not at goal in spite of three or more drugs of different pharmacologic classes being administered in appropriate doses with diuretics being at least one of the drug classes. Individuals who are obese are at high risk for resistant hypertension; >40% of patients who have resistant hypertension are obese. As compared to lean patients, obese patients need a more number of agents, as well as greater doses of medication for achieving control.

Levels of circulating leptin and insulin are reduced by weight loss. Reduction in weight partially reverses resistance to both hormones, reduces sympathetic activation, reduces activity of plasma renin and levels of aldosterone, and improves BP as well as other risk factors for atherosclerosis. A meta-analysis reported that significant weight loss attained by dietary interventions can reduce BP. With every kilogram of reduction in weight, it has been shown that weight loss reduces BP by 0.3 mm Hg. Reduction in weight should be considered as a primary treatment goal as obesity may add to metabolic as well as cardiovascular risks associated with hypertension. In addition to this, reduction in weight may result in improvement of hypertension-associated organ damage (reduction in excretion of urinary protein and left ventricular mass) independently of BP.

Recently, two novel drugs have been approved by FDA in addition to a decreased calorie diet and increase in physical activity for management of chronic weight in case of overweight (with BMI 27) or obese adults (with BMI 30) having minimum one weight-related coexisting condition such as hypertension, T2DM, increased cholesterol or sleep apnea. These two new drugs are lorcaserin, which is a selective agonist of the serotonin receptor, and phentermine plus extended release topiramate, which is a fixed-dose combination of an anorectic agent and an antiepileptic drug. Trials have shown favorable changes in blood pressure and cardiovascular risk factors, however long-term side effects and long-term cardiovascular safety need to be assessed.

There is an increase in use of bariatric surgery as a therapeutic alternative for controlling obesity. Laparoscopic sleeve gastrectomy resolves or improves hypertension in nearly 75% of patients, however no long-term effect on the incidence of hypertension is noted.

The mechanisms that are involved in arterial hypertension associated with obesity are that obesity-associated arterial hypertension comes with volume expansion and increases neurohumoral activation. The reasonable first choices include renin–angiotensin system inhibitors, diuretics, and beta-blockers. In majority of the patients, first-line antihypertensives are the inhibitors of the renin–angiotensin system. Currently, ACE inhibitors are the most appropriate drugs in such patients due to their broad spectrum of beneficial effects. In the patients who cannot tolerate angiotensin-converting enzyme inhibition, angiotensin II receptor blockers can be utilized. Even though renin–angiotensin system inhibitors may be the first choice antihypertensive, monotherapy is seldom sufficient to control blood pressure. More than 50% of the obese patients with hypertension are treated with two or more antihypertensive drugs in the primary care setting.

Cardiac output and renin activity, frequently increased in obese patients, are reduced by beta-blockers. As compared to lean hypertensive individuals, in obese individuals, beta-blockers alone are more effective in reducing BP. In younger obese hypertensive patients who do not have cardiac and renal complications, limitations for the usage of beta-blockers include their potential negative effects on glucose metabolism as well as body weight. Vasodilating beta-blockers with alpha-blocking activity, e.g., carvedilol, nebivolol, etc., seem to be lacking this negative metabolic profile, which is potentially associated with their better peripheral glucose disposal effects permitted by vasodilatory component of these drugs. However, their effectiveness has not been determined in improvement of cardiovascular outcomes in obesity-related hypertension.

With respect to the well-known hypervolemia and sodium retention in obesity, diuretic agents are utilized. Thiazide diuretics are more commonly used with renin-angiotensin-aldosterone system (RAAS) inhibitors for better blood pressure control. High-dose thiazide diuretics are associated with impaired glucose metabolism and insulin sensitivity which are already impaired in centrally obese patients. In majority of the obese hypertensive patients, thiazide diuretics may not be considered as the first choice. However, these are believed to be a reasonable second or third antihypertensive drug among patients who do not respond to monotherapy.

The dihydropyridine calcium-channel blockers are known to be effective in reducing BP. One of the potential limitations is the finding that as compared to lean patients, obese patients are more likely to develop peripheral edema with treatment with dihydropyridine calcium channel blocker.

In the management of resistant hypertension in case of obese individuals, aldosterone antagonist plays a special role. A study included true resistant hypertension patients who were diagnosed by ambulatory blood pressure monitoring (ABPM). Patients received spironolactone treatment in doses of 25 mg was performed after a median interval of 7 months, which showed a reduction of 16/9 mm Hg in BP. Outstandingly, higher waist circumference was found to be associated with better response to spironolactone. There is no existence of such data for eplerenone; however, it can be an effective option in patients who have adverse effects from spironolactone.

In obese hypertensive patients, an effective alternative treatment approach is direct renin inhibition. They should be not be used in combination with other renin-angiotensin system inhibitors or renal disease in view of risk of hyperkalemia. It has not been shown to have improvement in primary cardiovascular and renal outcomes.

The treatment of obesity-related hypertension seems to be mechanistically attractive. However, in clinical practice, due to the adverse effects (e.g., sedation) and inferior outcomes, the effects of sympatholytic drugs (such as clonidine or α-methyldopa) are disappointing. With novel imidazoline agonists, these side effects appear less prominently. They have similar efficacy to hydrochlorothiazide and angiotensin converting enzyme inhibitors. Moxonidine was also noted to induce a 1- to 2-kg weight loss and to improve insulin sensitivity. These drugs lack the support from clinical outcome trials. Use of moxonidine in heart failure patients has been found to be associated with increase in mortality because of the worsening of heart failure.

Renal sympathetic denervation and baroreflex activation therapy are under investigation and have shown to be effective in resistant hypertension in obese people. In baroreflex activation therapy, surgical implantation of an electrical stimulatory device as well as electrodes positioned at the carotid sinus level is required. Renal sympathetic denervation through a novel catheter-based approach and electrical stimulation of carotid baroreceptor approaches need to be investigated in large scale clinical trials in the near future.

SUGGESTED READING

1. Grassi G. How to treat hypertension in the obese? ESC. 2013;12(2).
2. Kidambi S, Kotchen TA. Treatment of hypertension in obese patients. Am J Cardiovasc Drugs. 2013;13(3):163-75.
3. Landsberg L, Aronne LJ, Beilin LJ, et al. Obesity-related hypertension: pathogenesis, cardiovascular risk, and treatment: a position paper of The Obesity Society and the American Society of Hypertension. J Clin Hypertens (Greenwich). 2013;15(1):14-33.

CASE 5: Hypertension in Smokers

A 60-year-old gentleman who is a retired bank employee came to OPD with complaints of occasional cough with expectoration. He told that he is a smoker, taking 10 cigarettes per day (moderate smoker), and takes minimal alcohol. No other cardiovascular risk factors are present. In spite of taking into consideration nonpharmacological advice of increase in exercise and restricting intake of salt, his average blood pressure was 160/100 mm Hg from several readings taken over the last 4 months. He often skips his medicines.

On examination, his heart rate was 90 beats/min and blood pressure was 170/100 mm Hg. Cardiovascular examination was essentially normal. His blood investigations, ECG, and echocardiography were done on OPD basis.

Blood reports showed random blood sugar of 160 mg%, blood urea of 59 mg/dL, and serum creatinine of 1.8 mg%.

An electrocardiogram revealed changes suggestive of left ventricular hypertrophy (LVH). Chest X-ray was suggestive of features of chronic obstructive pulmonary disease (COPD).

Baseline echocardiography showed LVH, with septal and posterior wall thickness of 14 mm, and an LV end-diastolic dimension of 4.5 cm, with left ventricular ejection fraction (LVEF) of 60%. His resting pulmonary artery systolic pressure (PASP) was 30 mm Hg.

Q1. Cigarette smoking causes atherothrombotic process by which of the following mechanisms?
   a. Impairment of endothelial function
   b. Inflammation and lipid modification

c. Alteration of antithrombotic and prothrombotic factors
d. All of the above

Q2. Which of the following statements is incorrect?
a. There was an average elevation in systolic pressure of 20 mm Hg after the first cigarette smoke
b. The adrenergic involvement in the acute hemodynamic effect of smoking is explained by peripheral mechanism (that includes stimulation of adrenal gland, norepinephrine reuptake reduction, catecholamine clearance reduction, etc.) instead of central mechanisms
c. There is inhibition of central sympathetic drive instead of excitation possibly due to arterial baroreceptor stimulation
d. None of the above

Q3. Which of the following statements is correct?
a. Smoking cigarettes causes arterial stiffness that can endure for a decade following cessation of smoking
b. As observed in some of the studies, habitual smokers usually have reduced blood pressures as compared to nonsmokers
c. Cotinine is the major metabolite of nicotine and its vasodilator effect may lead to the reduced BP
d. All of the above

Q4. Which of the following statements is incorrect?
a. Acute smoking of one cigarette induced acute increases of heart rate, brachial blood pressure, and aortic pulse wave velocity
b. Passive or environmental smoking is not associated with acute deterioration in aortic stiffness
c. Chronic smokers had higher augmentation index as compared to nonsmokers
d. Cigarette smoking might affect preferentially central blood pressure, by increasing arterial stiffness and wave reflection

Q5. Which of the following statements is incorrect?
a. Left ventricular mass was greater in the smokers than in the nonsmokers
b. Atherosclerotic disease in smokers develops approximately 10 years earlier than in nonsmokers
c. Smoking enhances the progression of renal insufficiency
d. Cessation of smoking can rapidly lower the risk of coronary heart disease by 15–20%

Ans. 1-d, 2-d, 3-d, 4-b, 5-d

HYPERTENSION IN SMOKERS

The most common cause of avoidable cardiovascular mortality, across the globe, is the use of tobacco. Presently, there are 1.3 billion cigarette smokers; out of which 82% are from developing countries. An estimated 1 billion deaths related to

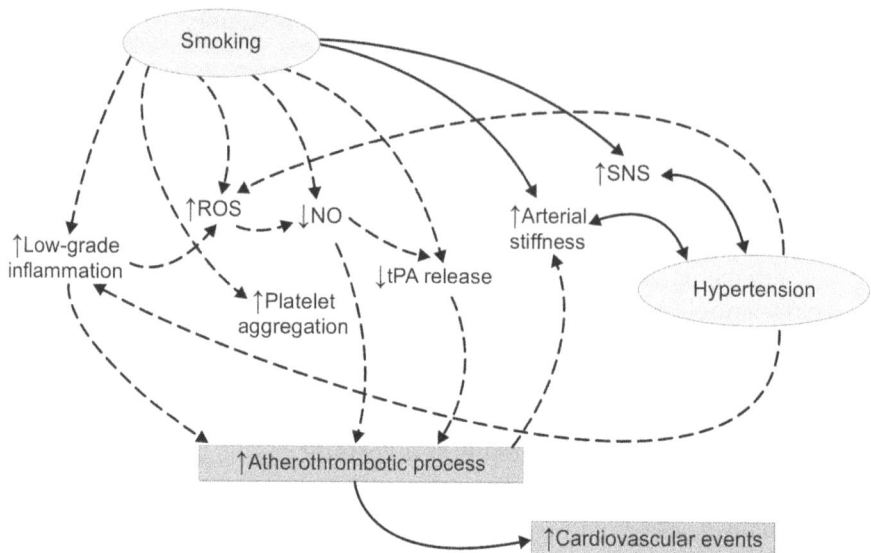

(NO: nitric oxide; ROS: reactive oxygen species; SNS: sympathetic nervous III system; tPA: tissue plasminogen activator)

Fig. 1: Schematic representation of the main mechanisms whereby smoking, hypertension (broken lines), and their association (continuous lines), can facilitate and accelerate the atherothrombotic process. See text for further explanations.

tobacco use will occur during the 21st century, if the current practices continue. The immediate noxious effects of smoking are associated with sympathetic nervous overactivity. This enhances consumption of myocardial oxygen via an increase in blood pressure, heart rate as well as myocardial contractility.

Smoking of cigarette predisposes a person to many different clinical atherosclerotic syndromes, which comprise of acute coronary syndromes, stable angina, stroke, and aortic and peripheral atherosclerosis, resulting in abdominal aortic aneurysm as well as intermittent claudication. Major determinants of initiation, promotion as well as precipitation of the atherothrombotic process include endothelial function impairment, inflammation, lipid modification, and an alteration of antithrombotic and prothrombotic factors. This is summarized in **Figure 1**.

EFFECT OF CIGARETTE SMOKING ON BLOOD PRESSURE AND HYPERTENSION

Acute Effects of Smoking on Blood Pressure

Smoking cigarette is identified to be accompanied by an acute rise in blood pressure and heart rate. It is reported by studies that heavy smoking is related to an increase in blood pressure, which remains for >15 minutes following smoking one cigarette, and along with a rise in blood pressure variability. As reported by some studies, there is an association between acute increase in blood pressure and heart rate (induced by cigarette smoking) and an increase in plasma catecholamines. This suggests that the effect is mediated by the adrenergic nervous system stimulation. However, a concomitant specular reduction is shown by sympathetic nerve activity. Therefore, peripheral (which includes stimulation of adrenal gland, decrease in reuptake of norepinephrine, catecholamine clearance reduction, etc.) instead of central mechanisms describe the adrenergic involvement in the acute hemodynamic effect of smoking, because there is inhibition of central sympathetic drive instead of excitation possibly due to stimulation of arterial baroreceptor.

There is an increase in blood pressure transiently with each cigarette. In cases where the blood pressure is taken 30 minutes after the last smoke, the pressor effect may be missed. Even in habitual smokers, the transient increase in blood pressure may be most prominent after smoking first cigarette of the day. According to a study that included normotensive smokers, an average increase in systolic blood pressure of 20 mm Hg was observed after smoking the first cigarette (**Fig. 1**). Moreover, in patients with mild primary hypertension (previously known as "essential" hypertension), ambulatory blood pressure monitoring indicates an interactive effect between smoking and drinking coffee, which leads to a mean increase in daytime systolic blood pressure of nearly 6 mm Hg.

Chronic Effects of Smoking on Blood Pressure

Cigarette smoking chronically leads to arterial stiffness that can remain for a decade after cessation of smoking. In the individuals who smoke 15 or more cigarettes per day, the incidence of hypertension is increased. In asymptomatic people, the coexistence of hypertension and smoking reduces left ventricular function.

However, as compared to nonsmokers, habitual smokers usually have reduced blood pressure as noted in almost majority of the studies. In smokers, the mild decrease in blood pressure is associated with reduction in body weight. What supports this finding is the increased body weight and blood pressure in former smokers in comparison to that noted in never-smokers. Cotinine, the main metabolite of nicotine, can also lead to lower blood pressure by its vasodilator effect.

Smoking, Central Blood Pressure, and Arterial Stiffness

Smoking can affect the brachial and central blood pressure in different ways. In smokers, acute cigarette smoking was observed to elevate carotid or aortic stiffness. More recently, it has been observed that in both nonsmokers and chronic smokers, acute cigarette smoking increases central blood pressure and parameters of arterial stiffness as well as peripheral wave reflection.

The greatest effects of short-term smoking on arterial stiffness seem to occur in the first 5 minutes after smoking. The magnitude of increase in arterial stiffness following smoking was comparable among nonsmokers and smokers. Acute smoking of one cigarette (having nicotine content 0.9 mg) by hypertensive

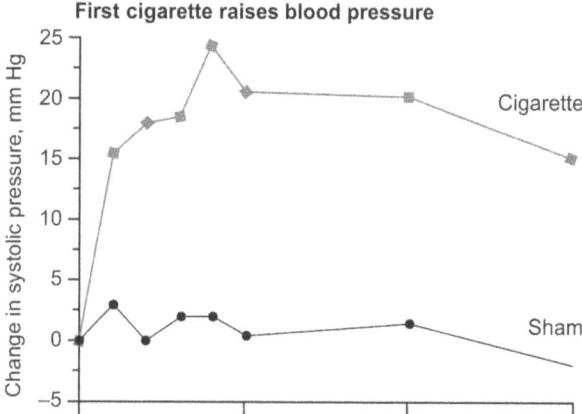

Fig. 2: Change in systolic blood pressure over 15 minutes after smoking the first cigarette of the day (squares) or during sham smoking (circles) in 10 normotensive smokers. Smoking was associated with a 15–20 mm Hg rise in systolic pressure that began to dissipate at 15 minutes.

Source: Adapted from Groppelli A, Giorgi DM, Omboni S, et al. Persistent blood pressure increase induced by heavy smoking. J Hypertens. 1992;10(5):495-9.

male smokers leads to acute increases in heart rate, brachial blood pressure, and aortic pulse wave velocity (PWV) in normotensives comparable to hypertensives. In hypertensive patients, however, the effect remained for a longer time (up to 15 min) and increase in PWV was significant following adjustment for heart rate and brachial mean arterial pressure. Passive or environmental smoking is also found to be related to acute deterioration in aortic stiffness (which is measured with the aortic pressure diameter loop), which increased within 4 minutes of passive smoking, similar to active smokers.

In a limited number of healthy individuals or hypertensive patients, the chronic effects of smoking on brachial and central blood pressure have been evaluated. In a study, 41 normotensive chronic smokers matched for age, gender, height, and weight were compared with 116 nonsmokers. It was found that chronic smokers had higher central systolic blood pressure and augmentation index as compared to nonsmokers (**Fig. 2**). While chronic smokers had reduced aortic-brachial pulse pressure amplification, in spite of a similar brachial blood pressure.

To conclude, smoking cigarette can especially have an effect on central blood pressure, by causing increase in arterial stiffness as well as wave reflection. The adverse effect of smoking on CV damage could be mediated by this phenomenon. However, future studies evaluating the impact of cessation of smoking on arterial stiffness and central blood pressure should support this hypothesis.

SMOKING-MEDIATED TARGET ORGAN DAMAGE AND HYPERTENSION SYNDROMES

Verdecchia et al. studied the relationship between cigarette smoking and left ventricular mass. They observed that following adjustment for clinic blood pressure and other related covariates, left ventricular mass resulted greater in the smokers than in the nonsmokers.

Smoking speeds up atheromas, particularly at the levels of carotid, intracerebral as well as coronary arteries. Smokers develop atherosclerotic disease about 10 years earlier than nonsmokers.

Many retrospective studies reported that hypertensive smokers are more likely to develop renovascular hypertension. Renal artery stenosis related to smoking is mostly atherosclerotic. Clinician should have a particular suspicion of a renovascular hypertension when in front to a cigarette smoker patient, especially if other typical clinical features occur, including onset of hypertension over the age of 60 years, or stage 3 or 4 hypertension in young patients, refractory hypertension, coronary or peripheral vascular disease.

Progression of renal insufficiency is increased by smoking. In a prospective study (that had a mean follow-up of 35 months), example of the latter effect was noted. In that study, the factors associated with alterations in renal function were examined in 53 hypertensive patients which had serum creatinine levels increased from 1.5–1.9 mg/dL (133–168 μmol/L) in spite of a significant decrease in the target mean blood pressure (from 127 mm Hg to 97 mm Hg). The most significant independent factor underlying progressive renal disease was smoking [serum creatinine 1.5 mg/dL and 2.1 mg/dL (133 μmol/L and 186 μmol/L) at the starting and end of the study for smokers, respectively, vs. 1.25 mg/dL and 1.32 mg/dL (110 μmol/L and 117 μmol/L) for nonsmokers, respectively]. The mechanism that exists behind this adverse effect is still not clear but it may be associated with the transient rise in systemic blood pressure with smoking being transmitted to the glomerulus, leading to glomerular hypertension.

The malignant hypertension is the other frequent form of hypertension syndrome that characterizes hypertensive smoker patients. In particular, it was noted that, as compared to nonsmokers, hypertensive smokers are found to be five times more likely to develop malignant hypertension.

Smoking cessation will rapidly reduce the risk of coronary heart disease by 35–40%. This effect is independent of the smoking duration. It is not known if smoking cessation has a similar benefit in preserving renal function.

KEY POINTS

- There is a transient increase in blood pressure with each cigarette; if the blood pressure is measured 30 minutes following the last smoke, the pressor effect may be missed. Even in habitual smokers, the transient rise in blood pressure may be the most prominent with the first cigarette of the day.
- As compared to nonsmokers, habitual smokers usually have reduced blood pressure. In smokers, the mild decrease in blood pressure is associated with reduction in body weight. Cotinine is the major metabolite of nicotine. It may also lead to the reduced blood pressure by vasodilator effect.
- In patients with hypertension, it is recommended to avoid smoking as it can significantly enhance the risk of secondary cardiovascular complications as well as increase the progression of renal insufficiency.

SUGGESTED READING

1. Najem B, Houssière A, Pathak A, et al. Acute cardiovascular and sympathetic effects of nicotine replacement therapy. Hypertension. 2006;47(6):1162-7.
2. Deanfield JE, Halcox JP, Rabelink TJ. Endothelial function and dysfunction: testing and clinical relevance. Circulation. 2007;115(10):1285-95.
3. Grassi G, Seravalle G, Calhoun DA, et al. Mechanisms responsible for sympathetic activation by cigarette smoking in humans. Circulation 1994;90(1):248-53.
4. Groppelli A, Giorgi DM, Omboni S, et al. Persistent blood pressure increase induced by heavy smoking. J Hypertens. 1992;10(5):495-9.
5. Jatoi NA, Jerrard-Dunne P, Feely J, et al. Impact of smoking and smoking cessation on arterial stiffness and aortic wave reflection in hypertension. Hypertension. 2007;49(5):981-5.
6. Primatesta P, Falaschetti E, Gupta S, et al. Association between smoking and blood pressure: evidence from the health survey for England. Hypertension. 2001;37(2):187-93.
7. Rhee MY, Na SH, Kim YK, et al. Acute effects of cigarette smoking on arterial stiffness and blood pressure in male smokers with hypertension. Am J Hypertens. 2007;20(6):637-41.
8. Verdecchia P, Schillaci G, Borgioni C, et al. Cigarette smoking, ambulatory blood pressure and cardiac hypertrophy in essential hypertension. J Hypertens. 1995;13(10):1209-15.
9. Regalado M, Yang S, Wesson DE. Cigarette smoking is associated with augmented progression of renal insufficiency in severe essential hypertension. Am J Kidney Dis. 2000;35(4):687-94.

SECTION 2
Hypertension – Types

YP Munjal

CASE 1: Resistant Hypertension

A 55-year-old woman, known hypertensive since past 6 years, came to OPD with complaints of persistent headache. She denied any history of chest pain, dyspnea, or visual disturbance. On examination, the heart rate (HR) was 64 bpm and blood pressure was 180/100 mm Hg. Cardiovascular system (CVS) and respiratory system (RS) examinations were clinically normal. Electrocardiogram (ECG) showed left ventricular hypertrophy (LVH). She had been compliant with her medication which included 10 mg amlodipine, 100 mg atenolol, and 12.5 mg chlorthalidone.

Q1. Resistant hypertension is defined as all these, as per Indian Guidelines on Hypertension IV recommendations, except
   a. Not able to attain BP <140/90 mm Hg
   b. 2 drugs + 1 diuretic at maximum tolerable dose
   c. 3 drugs + 1 diuretic at maximum tolerable dose
   d. Does not include newly detected case of systemic hypertension

Q2. The prevalence of resistant hypertension is around:
   a. <1%
   b. 20–25%
   c. 70–75%
   d. 85–90%

Q. 3. All these are termed as "pseudo-resistance", except:
   a. Suboptimal BP recording techniques
   b. Thick walled arteries in elderly (Osler's sign)
   c. White coat effect
   d. Poor adherence to antihypertensive drugs

Q4. The risk factors associated with resistant hypertension:
   a. Diabetes
   b. Left ventricular hypertrophy
   c. Black race
   d. All

Q5. Nonsteroidal anti-inflammatory drugs (NSAIDs) cause resistant hypertension due to which mechanism:
   a. Inhibit prostacyclin synthesis
   b. Decrease renal blood flow

c. Sodium and water retention
d. All of the above

Ans. 1-c, 2-b, 3-b, 4-d, 5-d

DISCUSSION

Resistant hypertension is defined as blood pressure that remains above goal of <140/90 mm Hg in spite of the use of three antihypertensive agents of different classes. One of the three agents should be a diuretic. All the agents should be prescribed in optimal doses. What constitutes an "optimal dose" of medication is a moderate dose but not necessarily a maximum dose.

PREVALENCE AND PROGNOSIS

The exact prevalence of resistant hypertension in the general population remains unknown. Data from different studies shows a wide variation from 10% to 30% in different populations.

"Uncontrolled hypertension" is not resistant hypertension. This includes patients who lack blood pressure control due to poor adherence and/or an inadequate treatment regimen. Patients with true resistant hypertension are part of it also.

The prognosis of resistant hypertension is worse than those with good blood pressure control. Patients with secondary hypertension often have resistant hypertension unless the underlying cause is treated. We should investigate patients with resistant hypertension more extensively for secondary causes. Also, they more often have associated cardiovascular risk factors such as diabetes, obstructive sleep apnea, left ventricular hypertrophy (LVH), and/or chronic kidney disease (CKD).

True and pseudo-resistant hypertension, it is important to determine whether the hypertension is truly resistant.

True resistant hypertension includes those who have uncontrolled clinic and home blood pressures despite being compliant with an antihypertensive regimen that includes three or more drugs.

Pseudo-resistant hypertension includes patients with uncontrolled blood pressure that is due to factors other than true resistance. This may be due to white-coat effect, suboptimal doses, lack of compliance, or concomitant use of drugs such as NSAIDs or alcohol.

Patient Characteristics Associated with Resistant Hypertension

- Older age
- High baseline blood pressure
- Obesity
- Excessive dietary salt ingestion
- Chronic kidney disease

- Diabetes
- Left ventricular hypertrophy
- Black race
- Female sex
- Residence in southeastern United States.

A variety of medications can raise the blood pressure and, in some cases, reduce the response to antihypertensive drugs. These include:
- *Non-narcotic analgesics:*
  - Nonsteroidal anti-inflammatory agents, including aspirin
  - Selective cyclooxygenase-2 (COX-2) inhibitors
- Sympathomimetic agents (decongestants, diet pills, and cocaine)
- Stimulants (dextroamphetamine, amphetamine, and modafinil)
- Alcohol
- Oral contraceptives
- Cyclosporine
- Erythropoietin
- Natural licorice
- Herbal compounds (ephedra)

Secondary causes: Patients with resistant hypertension are also much more likely to have an identifiable cause of hypertension.

Common:
- Obstructive sleep apnea
- Renal parenchymal disease
- Primary aldosteronism
- Renal artery stenosis

Uncommon:
- Pheochromocytoma
- Cushing's disease
- Hyperparathyroidism
- Aortic coarctation
- Intracranial tumor

EVALUATION

The evaluation should be directed toward confirmation of true resistance; identification of causes contributing to resistance, secondary causes of hypertension; and evaluation of target-organ damage. Blood pressure measurements should be done at home and in the clinic both. In some cases, ambulatory BP monitoring may be required.

Medical history for duration, severity and progression of the blood pressure; treatment adherence, response to prior medications, adverse effects of drugs, and current medications must be evaluated. History of use of herbal, over-the-counter medications, and other drugs known to increase BP such as cocaine, amphetamines, cyclosporine, tacrolimus, tobacco, and some illicit drugs. History pointing toward secondary causes of hypertension should be taken. Drug compliance at times depends on cost factors, which needs to be looked at. At times patients miss drugs when they have other concomitant acute ailments.

Usual precautions for proper BP measurement technique should be adopted. This includes having the patient sit quietly in a chair with his or her back supported for 5 minutes before taking the measurement; use of the correct cuff size with the air bladder encircling at least 80% of the arm. The arm should be at heart level during the measurement. Minimum of 3 readings should be taken at intervals of at least 1 minute and the average of those readings should be taken.

The white coat effect can be assessed by comparing home blood pressure measurement (HBPM) with the office blood pressure values. Multiple readings should be undertaken in both settings. More recently automated office blood pressure (AOBP) can be used since it partly eliminated the white coat effect. AOBP readings are often less than physician/nurse measured manual blood pressure office readings although they are often somewhat higher than the HBPM readings. At times of 24-hour ambulatory blood pressure monitoring may be done.

Biochemical evaluation of resistant hypertensive should include routine metabolic profile (sodium, potassium, glucose, blood urea nitrogen, and creatinine) and urine analysis. Plasma aldosterone levels to look for primary aldosteronism should be done. Once biochemical parameters are suggestive of a secondary cause imaging can be used. Ultrasound abdomen and renal Doppler studies are cost effective and can be used initially. Computed tomography (CT) abdomen for adrenal masses or renal pathology and radio nuclear imaging are to be used where initial imaging studies or biochemistry raises suspicion of secondary causes.

■ TREATMENT RECOMMENDATIONS

- Maximize the drug adherence.
- Nonpharmacological recommendations should be emphasized. This includes weight loss, dietary salt restriction, moderation of alcohol intake, increased physical activity, and ingestion of a high-fiber and low-fat diet.
- Treatment of secondary causes of hypertension whenever diagnosed.

Better BP control is achieved by combining drugs from different classes rather than by increasing the dose of a single medication. Use multiple drugs in combination. Pill burden should be kept low by using fixed dose combinations.

Aldosterone-antagonist spironolactone should be added as the fourth agent once angiotensin-converting enzyme inhibitor/angiotensin receptor blocker (ACE inhibitor/ARB) + calcium channel blocker (CCB) and thiazide like diuretic has been used. The PATHWAY 2 study showed that it is to be preferred over beta-blockers and doxazosin as an add on therapy. Therapy with mineralocorticoid receptor antagonist involves pharmacologic blockade of the mineralocorticoid receptor targeting the excess aldosterone commonly present in patients with resistant hypertension (RH). Spironolactone is most frequently used. Eplerenone has fewer adverse effects but is a costlier and less potent alternative. Spironolactone may reduce systolic BP by 15–20 mm Hg in patients with hypertension that is resistant to 3 drugs.

Further add on agents for those in whom blood pressure is still uncontrolled can include vasodilating β-blocker (e.g., labetalol, carvedilol, and nebivolol), direct vasodilators (e.g., hydralazine or centrally acting agent such as clonidine) or alpha methyldopa.

Recent technological advances, along with the growing need for effective management of RH, rekindled the concept of interventional management and made it one of the hottest research areas in hypertension. Interventional options available are carotid baroreceptor activation and renal denervation.

A small device, like a pacemaker, is used to constantly activate carotid baroreceptors. The effects of carotid baroreceptor activation are mediated by the attenuation of sympathetic nervous activity. Muscle sympathetic nervous activity (MSNA), a reliable and commonly used index of systemic SNA, has been shown to be reduced following baroreceptor activation. Long-term efficacy and outcome data from large randomized controlled trials (RCTs) are needed to establish baroreceptor activation as a viable alternative for the management of RH.

Renal denervation therapy using radiofrequency probes to ablate the sympathetic fibers along the renal artery showed great promise in initial studies. The SYMPLICITY 1 and 2 studies showed reduction in BP with renal denervation. These results were better than the drug therapy. However, the subsequent larger and more meticulous study, the SYMPLICITY 3 trial showed that there was no significant difference in patient outcome between renal denervation and a sham procedure among patients with drug resistant hypertension. After 6 months, office systolic blood pressure decreased from baseline to a similar extent in the renal-denervation and sham-procedure groups. These findings contradict most published data on renal denervation.

SUGGESTED READINGS

1. Calhoun DA, Jones D, Textor S, et al. Resistant hypertension: Diagnosis, evaluation, and treatment: A scientific statement from the American Heart Association Professional Education Committee of the Council for High Blood Pressure Research. Circulation. 2008;117:e51026.
2. Myat A, Redwood SR, Qureshi AC, et al. Resistant hypertension. BMJ. 2012;345:e7473.
3. Viera AJ. Resistant hypertension. J Am Board Fam Med. 2012;25:487-95.
4. Vongpatanasin W. Resistant hypertension—a review of diagnosis and management. JAMA. 2014;311(21):2216-24.

CASE 2: Isolated Systolic Hypertension

A 72-year-old gentleman, retired government officer, presented in the OPD. He is in good health. There is no significant medical history in the past except for an uneventful inguinal hernia surgery 10 years back. He has no other cardiac risk factor such as diabetes, smoking, obesity, or dyslipidemia. A routine health check-up for senior citizen revealed a blood pressure (BP) of 180/80 mm Hg. He does "brisk walks" regularly in the morning for 30 minutes, at least 5 days a week. Clinical examination revealed short systolic murmur over the aortic area. Baseline biochemical investigations, including renal function were normal. Lipid profile was normal. Electrocardiogram (ECG) showed evidence of left ventricular hypertrophy. ECG showed aortic valve sclerosis with no hemodynamically significant transaortic gradient or regurgitation. A clinical diagnosis of isolated systolic hypertension (ISH) was made. Therapy was initiated with a combination of calcium channel blocker (CCB—amlodipine) with low dose diuretic (chlorthalidone).

Q1. Individual with blood pressure recording of 172/84 mm Hg should be classified as?
 a. High normal
 b. Isolated systolic hypertension
 c. Grade 1 hypertension
 d. Grade 2 hypertension

Q2. About ISH, which of the following statement is not true?
 a. Raised systolic pressure with normal or low diastolic pressure is seen
 b. Widened pulse pressure is observed
 c. It is a disease of elderly
 d. Need not to be treated with antihypertensive therapy

Q3. Which of the following statements is wrong regarding management of ISH?
 a. Lifestyle modification rarely helps
 b. Thiazide diuretics can be used as first line drug
 c. In patients with benign prostatic hyperplasia (BPH), one can use alpha blocking agents
 d. All of the above statements are wrong

Q4. All is true regarding lifestyle modifications for management, except:
 a. Dietary sodium restriction
 b. Physical exercise
 c. Low fiber diet
 d. Moderation of alcohol

Q5. Which of the following is/are risk factor for development of ISH?
   a. Cigarette smoking
   b. Alcohol abuse
   c. Diabetes
   d. All of the above

Ans. 1-b, 2-d, 3-a, 4-c, 5-d

DISCUSSION

Isolated systolic hypertension is seen more often in the elderly. Systolic blood pressure (SBP) is known to rise with advancing age; whereas diastolic BP usually levels off and does not change beyond 60 years. ISH is the most prevalent type of hypertension in those over 60 years of age and represents a substantial healthcare problem as the target BP is more difficult to attain. ISH is defined as systolic BP >140 mm Hg and diastolic BP <90 mm Hg.

CLASSIFICATION

ISH	Systolic (mm Hg)		Diastolic (mm Hg)
Stage 1	140–159	and	<90
Stage 2	>160	and	<90

ETIOLOGY AND PATHOPHYSIOLOGY

Besides increase with advancing age, ISH may be seen in young patients. ISH in young individuals is seen especially among those who are obese and smokers. Subjects with hyperthyroidism, hyperaldosteronism, renal insufficiency and failure, and renal artery stenosis also have predominant systolic BP elevation. Similarly drug-induced hypertension [nonsteroidal anti-inflammatory drugs (NSAIDS), cyclooxygenase-2 (COX-2) inhibitors, corticosteroids, and cyclosporine], excess alcohol use, obstructive sleep apnea (OSA), anemia, beriberi, Paget's disease, and some cancers can cause a relative high output state resulting in greater systolic elevation.

Isolated systolic hypertension largely occurs due to progressive structural and functional changes in the arterial wall, involving endothelial dysfunction, atherosclerosis, aortic stiffness, increased wall stress, and pulse pressure. Vascular endothelial damage and mechanical strain from each stroke volume also play a role. Atherosclerosis progressively leads to the replacement of elastin by collagen and other structural proteins and the build of calcium in the arterial wall, and this in turn results in hypertrophy and fibrosis of arterial wall. All these factors lead to increased vascular stiffness and reduced compliance causing a decrease in the "Windkessel function" of the large arteries. Renin–angiotensin system also plays a role in the pathogenesis of arterial stiffness by decreasing elastin content and increasing collagen of arterial wall.

CLINICAL FEATURES

Isolated systolic hypertension is most often asymptomatic and diagnosed on routine examination. Severe hypertension or an abrupt rise of BP may cause headache, blurred vision, or dizziness. Epistaxis may be a presenting feature. Some patients may have concomitant end organ damage including symptoms of coronary artery disease (CAD), heart failure, arrhythmias, stroke, intermittent claudication due to peripheral arterial disease, aortic aneurysm, aortic dissection, features of hypertensive retinopathy, and renal insufficiency or failure.

EVALUATION

Evaluation should include assessment of other cardiovascular (CV) risk factors, potentially contributing lifestyle factors (diet, exercise, alcohol, smoking, body weight, and drugs), end organ damage and secondary causes of hypertension. Physical examination should include looking for all peripheral pulses, optic fundi, cardiac, and neurological system. Abdominal and carotid bruit should be looked for. Ambulatory BP Monitoring (ABPM) may be used in some elderly patients to identify white coat effect, nondippers, and to assess response to drugs. Home BP measurement (HBPM) should be advocated to all for monitoring the response to treatment. The devices are easily available and user friendly.

MANAGEMENT

The systolic BP is a stronger predictor of cerebrovascular and CV events than diastolic BP. Several intervention studies in ISH (such as SHEP, SYST-EUR, SYST-China, INSIGHT, and LIFE) have demonstrated beneficial effects of treatment of ISH. Effort should be made to bring down systolic BP below 140 mm Hg in all individuals. Patients with very low diastolic BP of below 60 mm Hg those who have known coronary artery disease one should keep in mind the J-curve phenomenon.

Lifestyle Changes

- *Weight reduction*: It improves insulin sensitivity, sleep apnea, and the response to drugs. It is advisable to maintain ideal body weight (BMI 18.5–24.9 kg/m^2).
- *Dietary sodium restriction:* Moderate degrees of sodium restriction to 2.4 g/day results in SBP reduction by 2–8 mm Hg. Indian diet contains 8–12 g of salt and it should be reduced to 5 g.
- *Diet changes:* Diet should be rich in fruits, vegetables, low in saturated and total fat, and high in fiber content. Besides better BP control, it helps in reducing the risk of CAD and stroke.
- *Moderation of alcohol:* Excessive alcohol use is a common cause of reversible hypertension. Binge alcohol use can be particularly harmful. Abstinence can cause systolic BP reduction of 4–6 mm Hg.
- *Avoidance of tobacco:* Smoking in any form including chewable tobacco is a significant contributory factor for ISH. Smoking cessation results in significant BP reduction.

- *Physical exercise*: Regular aerobic physical activity such as brisk walking at least 45 minutes daily for most of the days of the week results in SBP reduction by 4–8 mm Hg.
- *Stress management*: Relaxation techniques, yoga, and meditation can reduce BP. We should discourage excessive consumption of coffee.

Drug Treatment

Four major classes of antihypertensive agents can be used as first line drugs. These are: (1) diuretics, (2) CCBs, (3) angiotensin-converting enzyme (ACE) inhibitors, and (4) angiotensin receptor blockers (ARBs). Usual approach of combining ACE inhibitor/ARB with a diuretic or a CCB would be second step. As a third step all these three agents can be combined. Spironolactone is the fourth add on agent. In patients with symptoms of benign prosthetic hyperplasia, alpha-blockers like doxazosin or prazosin may be used early. Alpha-blockers can cause postural hypotension and so both lying and standing BP should be recorded.

The treatment algorithm for ISH can be as given below:

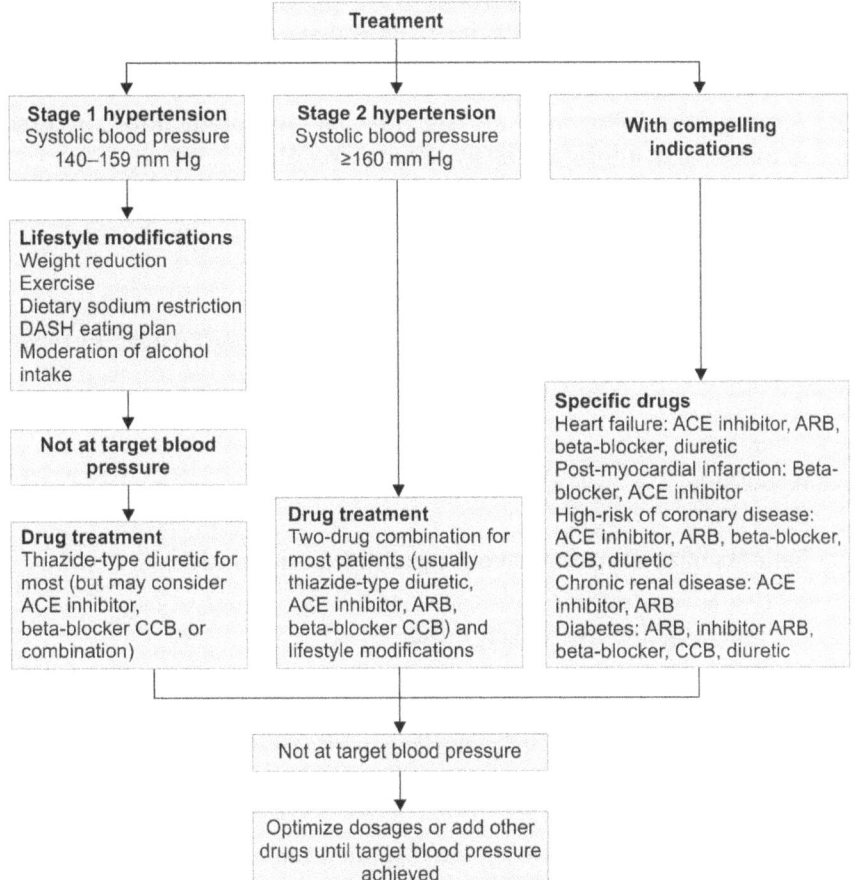

(ACE: angiotensin-converting enzyme; ARB: angiotensin receptor blockers; CCB: calcium channel blocker)

Flowchart 1: Treatment algorithm for patients with isolated systolic hypertension.

Isolated Systolic Hypertension in the Young

Isolated systolic hypertension among young adults is increasing in prevalence. Some patients with increased sympathetic activity can have tachycardia, features of anxiety and ISH. Isolated systolic hypertension in the young patients is often successfully treated with lifestyle modification and long-acting beta-blockers.

Obesity and smoking are also associated with ISH among young adults. Body fat has been shown to be a strong predictor of aortic stiffness in both young and older adults, which may account for the isolated elevation in SBP among obese young adults.

CASE 3: Downregulation of Antihypertensive Treatment

A 42-year-old male was diagnosed to have hypertension 3 years back. His hypertension has been well controlled and he has been having regular visits every 3 months. Presently he is taking tab amlodipine 5 mg once daily and is also compliant with dietary sodium restriction. He also exercises regularly, has lost 28 kg since past 3 years and presently weighs 78 kg. There is no evidence of any end-organ damage.

Q1. Among the following, all are the factors predicting successful withdrawal of antihypertensive drugs, except:
   a. Multiple antihypertensive drugs
   b. Lower doses of antihypertensive drugs
   c. Dietary compliance with sodium restriction
   d. Adherence to lifestyle modifications

Q2. What percentage of well-controlled stage I hypertensives to remain normotensive even after drug withdrawal?
   a. <15%
   b. 30–50%
   c. 50–80%
   d. >80%

Q3. Benefits of antihypertensive drug withdrawal include:
   a. Less adverse effects
   b. Better cognition, especially in elderly
   c. Both
   d. None

Q4. Possible mechanisms that make drug withdrawal successful:
   a. Blood pressure (BP) control may reverse hypertension-induced arteriolar hyperplasia
   b. Initial mislabeling of white-coat hypertension
   c. Failure to depend on lifestyle modifications initially
   d. All of the above

Q5. Withdrawal syndrome is characterized by:
  a. Decreased sympathetic activity
  b. Rebound hypertension
  c. Relief of angina
  d. All of the above

Ans. 1-a, 2-a, 3-c, 4-d, 5-b

DISCUSSION

Some patients with stage 1 hypertension are well controlled, often on a single medication. After a period of years, the question arises as to whether antihypertensive therapy can be gradually reduced or even discontinued. The issue of discontinuation of therapy also arises in patients who develop symptoms related to low blood pressure.

Selecting Patients for Antihypertensive Drug Downregulation

Antihypertensive treatment may be gradually reduced or discontinued in those patients who have mild hypertension and are well-controlled for a minimum duration of 1 year. Once treatment has been discontinued, 5–55% of patients stay normotensive for minimum 1-2 years. With a reduction in the number and/or dosage of medications taken, a larger number of patients do well.

As an example, as per a review that included published series of planned withdrawal, it was noted that 42% of the selected patients with mild hypertension (140-149/90-95 mm Hg) were found to remain normotensive for 12 months or longer off medication. Only 18% patients remained normotensive following discontinuation of medications in a more heterogeneous group of patients with well-controlled hypertension.

Patients who had milder hypertension, were taking fewer and lower doses of antihypertensive therapy, and were adherent to modifications in lifestyle (such as weight reduction and restriction of sodium) more likely tolerated cessation of antihypertensive therapy. It is suggested by these findings that in patients who are on multiple drugs, full withdrawal of antihypertensive medications may not be possible; however, gradual tapering of doses and agents of antihypertensive therapy may be possible.

The benefit of discontinuing successful drug therapy is still not certain, though lower doses are related to a lesser incidence of side effects induced by antihypertensive drugs. Therefore in well-controlled patients, it appears to be reasonable to decrease the dose, and withdraw if tolerated, with close monitoring of BP.

Observational studies have suggested that withdrawal of antihypertensive therapy in older adults with cognitive decline may improve cognitive function and prevent progression to dementia. However, a randomized trial found that discontinuation of antihypertensive therapy in older adults did not improve cognitive function. In this trial, 385 individuals who were 75 years or older with mild cognitive impairment, controlled hypertension (mean blood pressure 148/81 mm Hg), and no significant cardiovascular disease were assigned to have their antihypertensive therapy gradually discontinued or to have no changes made. At 16 weeks, blood pressure increased in the discontinuation group by 7/3 mm Hg, but there was no improvement in cognition or functional status.

Mechanism of Successful Drug Withdrawal

There is limited understanding of the mechanism of persistent normotension with less intensive drug treatment. Hypertension-induced arteriolar hyperplasia may be reversed with long-term BP control, thus decreasing vascular resistance directly as well as by decreasing the sensitivity to vasoconstrictors (e.g., angiotensin II and norepinephrine).

Medical Research Council trial studied this issue in a controlled fashion and gave an alternate explanation for this. The trial suggested that course of the disease may not be altered by effective therapy. But several patients being treated for mild hypertension are, in fact, normotensive or become normotensive by compliance with nonpharmacologic therapies. Many factors, specifically initial mislabeling and modifications in diet, can contribute to this effect. However, the ability to reduce drug dose in many patients may be because of the initial use of excessive dosage.

Mislabeling

Several patients who are initially diagnosed with mild hypertension are in fact normotensive. The increase in BP represents an acute stress response that is induced by visiting the clinician. This phenomenon, called "white coat" hypertension, illustrates the importance of repeated blood pressure measurements over several months in the office or, preferably, by multiple home measurements before considering an asymptomatic patient with no end-organ damage to be truly hypertensive. Sequential studies have shown that the blood pressure drops by an average of 10–15 mm Hg between the first and third office visits in newly diagnosed patients with mild hypertension, with a stable value not being achieved until >6 visits in some cases.

Dietary Modification

With the modifications in diet alone, initially hypertensive patients can reduce their BP to the normal range. While considering the step-down therapy, the triad of restriction of dietary sodium, weight loss in the obese person, and avoiding excess intake of alcohol may be especially significant. Persistent normotension following drug withdrawal may be most likely among nonobese patients who restrict sodium, and overweight patients who lose weight.

Excessive Doses

Now it is clear that for many antihypertensive drugs, previous dosing recommendations were too high. This resulted in a rise in incidence of side effects while yielding little if any further decrease in BP.

One final point needs to be highlighted. Abruptly discontinuing antihypertensive therapy with a short-acting alpha-2 agonist (such as clonidine) and a short-acting beta-blocker like propranolol can result in a potentially fatal withdrawal syndrome. This syndrome is characterized by rebound hypertension, enhanced sympathetic activity (because of upregulation of adrenergic receptor during the period of reduced sympathetic activity), as well as possible accelerated angina or myocardial infarction. For preventing this problem, these agents should be discontinued gradually over a period of weeks.

SUGGESTED READING

1. Mangrulkar S, Khair P, Hingne V, et al. Hypertension management and antihypertensive withdrawal: A perspective. JAPI. 2015;63(5):19-26.
2. Lemelin J. Does antihypertensive therapy need to be life-long. Can Fam Physician. 1989;35:1829-31.
3. Schmieder RE, Rockstroh JK, Messerli FH. Antihypertensive therapy. To stop or not to stop? JAMA. 1991;265(12):1566-71.

CASE 4: Poor Compliance in a Hypertensive

A 72-year-old hypertensive female came to emergency with complaints of sudden onset weakness of left side of the body with inability to talk since past 5 hours. She is a hypertensive on irregular medications. She had a history of insomnia and depression and a history of infrequent visit to the clinician. The family members could not give any details of her medications.

On examination, her heart rate was 66 beats/minute and blood pressure was 210/100 mm Hg. Respiratory rate was 18 breaths/minute. Cardiovascular examination was essentially normal with no S_3 or S_4. CNS examination showed left-sided complete hemiplegia with Broca's aphasia.

An electrocardiogram demonstrated left ventricular hypertrophy (LVH) with strain pattern. Baseline echocardiography showed normal LV systolic and type I diastolic dysfunction and no regional wall motion abnormalities. Urgent CT head was done and showed right middle cerebral artery (MCA) territory infarct.

Q1. Which of the following statements is correct?
  a. Ischemic stroke is the most common type of stroke in a hypertensive patient
  b. Hypertensive male >55 years of age and female >65 years are associated with increased cardiovascular risk
  c. Female age and depression are associated with poor adherence to medications
  d. All of the above

Q2. Measures to increase medication adherence in hypertension include all except:
   a. Low-dose combination therapy
   b. Fixed-dose single pill combination
   c. Frequent clinician visit and investigations to aware of complications
   d. Low-cost generics

Ans. 1-a, 2-c

DISCUSSION

Due to increased prevalence as well as its association with enhanced risk of cardiovascular disease, hypertension is considered to be one of the major health problems throughout the world. Hypertension can be defined as abnormally increased arterial blood pressure that includes elevated levels of systolic and/or diastolic blood pressure. It signifies persistent levels of systolic blood pressure ($\geq$140 mm Hg) and/or diastolic blood pressure ($\geq$90 mm Hg).

Problem in Hypertension Control

Despite the fact that there are constantly improving treatments available, only one-third of patients who are treated have a normalization of blood pressure. This is a worrying finding since it is proven that achieving normal blood pressure can reduce consequent neurological, cardiac, and vascular effects. One explanation of this lack of efficacy is undoubtedly poor therapeutic compliance with antihypertensive treatment.

Definition of Compliance

Compliance can be defined as the degree to which the patient conforms to medical advice about lifestyle and dietary changes as well as to keeping appointments for follow-up and taking treatment as prescribed. Compliance can be quantitatively defined as the percentage of prescribed doses that have been taken. At least 80% compliance is usually required in the treatment of hypertension for attaining an appropriate decrease in BP.

There are three components of compliance, which are:
1. Acceptance of prescribed medication.
2. Adherence to prescribed medication.
3. Continuation of prescribed medication.

Therefore, it can be stated that compliance is a health improving behavior that is complex and dynamic and includes actions such as appointment keeping, acquiring medicines and ingesting them, and persisting with health provider. Compliance with treatment at the individual level prevents complications and thus premature death, thereby improving the quality of life. It prevents the immediate family from having the negative psychological impact of living with or sudden death of a family member who suffers from a chronic debilitating disease (stroke). It also helps in conserving family resources, which would have been used for obtaining healthcare. Compliance with drug treatment in a larger society is an economical measure because it reduces the incidence of complications as well as the requirement for added medications. Health-related quality of life (HRQOL) stands for the physical, psychological, as well as social domains of health. It is the distinct areas that are affected by the experiences, beliefs, expectations, and perceptions of a person. Illness as well as treatment affects the perceptions of an individual about their quality of life. There are no symptoms in many patients with mild-to-moderate hypertension. Nonetheless, antihypertensive drug treatments are often related to unpleasant side effects that can affect other aspects of quality of life.

Methods of Evaluation of Compliance

The numerous methods of measurement of compliance can be divided into:
- *Pharmacological measures* (determination of serum and urinary concentrations of drugs or using biological markers integrated into the tablets).
- *Clinical measures* (clinical judgment of the doctor, evaluation of promptness for appointments or the use of questionnaires or taking the amount of side effects into account).
- *Physical measures* (verifying prescription renewals, counting the remaining pills or pill counting systems).

Pharmacological methods give percentages of noncompliance which are higher than found by other measures. They are generally thought to have a higher sensitivity and specificity but remain difficult to use in standard practice. Measurement of compliance by questioning the patient or counting remaining pills leads to overestimation of the number of tablets taken when compared to an electronic pill counting device.

To date, there is no gold standard allowing precise measurement of compliance. However, the electronic pill counter or Medication Event Monitoring System (MEMS) may be considered as the best existing system for measurement of compliance. This consists of a standard pillbox which has a microprocessor which can register the date and hour of the opening of the container. This helps in monitoring the amount of time between drug doses and the alteration in compliance with passage of time. However, cost as well as the correlation between opening drug container and compliance are among the many inconveniences.

Factors Influencing Compliance

There are four major determining influences on compliance:
1. The patient
2. The disorder
3. The treatment
4. The therapeutic environment

In a study conducted by Gallup, it was seen that 11% of patients treated with an antihypertensive stopped their treatment because of undesirable side effects, 25% because they thought that their doctor had asked them to, 46% because they thought they had been cured, and 6% for financial reasons.

The Patient
Significant factors associated with this context include the following:
- Social characteristics (age or social class) have little impact on the compliance of the patient.
- *Psychological characteristics*: Generally, hypertension is believed to be a result of anxiety, stress, or nervousness of the patient. So many believe that there is no need for treatment other than sedatives or anxiolytics.
- Furthermore some patients consider that this diagnosis is synonymous with the arrival of old age and thus reject the treatment.
- Depression is associated with poor control of hypertension.

The Disorder
There are no symptoms in majority of patients with hypertension. It is therefore hard to convince them to accept changes in treatment or lifestyle that prevent cardiac events in the long-term.

The Treatment
The undesirable effects of treatment are major obstacles to good compliance. The more frequent and handicapping they are, the less motivated the patient. In addition, in hypertension, these side effects occur in patients without clinical manifestations of their condition.

The Therapeutic Environment
The physician is accountable for the antihypertensive prescription. Compliance can be affected by the prescription due to its complexity; the more the number of antihypertensive medicines or tablets to be taken on daily basis, the less is the compliance.

Eisen et al., showed in a population of 105 hypertensive patients, that compliance went from 83.6% for a single daily dose to 59% for a three times a day dosage. The legibility of the prescription is also very important since this is generally the only written information given to the patient explaining how he should take the treatment.

As other healthcare professionals (pharmacists or nurses) are in special contact with the patient and usually the patient confides in them, they play an important role in compliance.

Improving Compliance
There are few unavoidable factors which may modify compliance; these include treatment duration or the absence of clinical signs related to the hypertension. Following are the means that could be used to improve compliance:
- *Detecting patients who are at risk*: As there are large errors in predicting such patients, this is very hard to achieve.
- Treatment can be optimized and simplified by using slow-release tablets and fixed combinations as much as possible and by prescribing the treatments that are best tolerated.

- Patients should be informed about their being hypertensive as well as about their treatment. The point to be kept in mind is that several patients are not familiar about the definition of hypertension and the normal blood pressure levels.
- Educating and involving patients so as to motivate and empower the person in order to make him aware of the necessity for treatment.
- Use of low-cost generics.
- Treatment of depression.

CONCLUSION

The major burden in control of hypertension is poor medication compliance. Increased age, female sex, depression, poor knowledge, and misconception regarding hypertension are major factors in poor medication compliance. Increased family and social support and more involvement of the treating physicians in information sharing to the patients and prescribing low cost, single dose effective generic medications will help to solve this problem and the severe consequences of this major cardiovascular disease.

SUGGESTED READING

1. Guerrero D, Rudd P, Bryant-Kosling C, et al. Antihypertensive medication-taking. Investigation of a simple regimen. Am J Hypertens. 1993;6(7):586-92.
2. Garfield FN, Caro JJ. Compliance and hypertension. Curr Hypertens Rep. 1999;1(6):502-6.
3. Eisen SA, Woodward RS, Miller D, et al. The effect of medication compliance on the control of hypertension. J Gen Intern Med. 1987;2(5):298-305.
4. Bailey BL, Carney SL, Gillies AH, et al. Hypertension treatment compliance: what do patients want to know about their medications? Prog Cardiovasc Nurs. 1997;12(4):23-8.

CASE 5: Hypertension and Wide Pulse Pressure

A 62-year-old man comes to OPD with frequent headaches over past 6 months. He has been known hypertensive since past 10 years, but poorly compliant with medications. He has no history of diabetes mellitus. His previous BP recordings are 150/100 mm Hg as told by the patient himself.

On examination, the heart rate was 102 beats/minute and blood pressure was 160/100 mm Hg. Cardiovascular examination was essentially normal. Blood reports showed random blood sugar: 270 mg%, blood urea: 59 mg/dL, and serum creatinine: 1.8 mg%.

Electrocardiogram revealed changes suggestive of left ventricular hypertrophy (LVH). Chest X-ray was within normal limits. Baseline echocardiography showed LVH, with septal and posterior wall thickness of 14 mm and an LV end-diastolic dimension of 4.5 cm, with left ventricular ejection fraction (LVEF) of 60%. His resting pulmonary artery systolic pressure (PASP) was 25 mm Hg.

Q1. Which of the following statements is incorrect?
   a. Pulse pressure is defined as the systolic minus the diastolic pressure
   b. After the age of 55 years, diastolic blood pressure declines on average
   c. A continuous increase in systolic pressure takes place with every decade of life; this helps in maintaining its predictive value for cardiovascular disease (CVD)
   d. Among the elderly, with increase in age, the pulse pressure does not correlate with the systolic blood pressure (SBP) than with the diastolic blood pressure (DBP), and therefore, it is not a good predictor of CVD

Q2. Which of the following statements is incorrect?
   a. In patients aged above 60 years, each 10 mm Hg increment in pulse pressure was associated with a 23% higher risk of developing coronary heart disease
   b. Higher pulse pressure is associated with an increased risk of developing diabetes
   c. A 10 mm Hg higher pulse pressure is associated with a 17% higher relative risk of developing ESRD
   d. None of above

Q3. Which of the following chromosome associations does not have a high degree of heritability with regard to increased pulse pressure?
   a. Chromosome 20
   b. Chromosome 19
   c. Chromosome 18
   d. Chromosome 17

Q4. Which of the following statements is correct?
   a. Shorter patients tend to have a higher pulse pressure
   b. Slower heart rates result in a greater pulse pressure
   c. Differences in pulse pressure with gender are lacking because the effect of height on pulse pressure may be counterbalanced by the effect of heart rate
   d. All of the above

Q5. Which of the following statements is incorrect?
   a. Increases in pulse pressure in older patients (e.g., >55 years of age) result from aortic stiffening
   b. Increases in younger patients (i.e., <45 years of age) are more likely to result from increase in stroke volume
   c. Diminished elastic recoil of aorta and an increased pressure decay rate cause a fall in the diastolic pressure with age
   d. None of the above

Ans. 1-d, 2-d, 3-a, 4-d, 5-d

INTRODUCTION

Typical BP measurements consist of a systolic and a diastolic value; this stands for the extremes of fluctuation in pressure in the circulation in the cardiac cycle. A lot of debate is going on regarding which increased value alone, either systolic or diastolic hypertension, is more predictive of adverse cardiovascular outcomes in various patient population.

CLINICAL PERSPECTIVE

Pulse pressure can be defined as the systolic pressure minus the diastolic pressure. In some of the epidemiologic studies, pulse pressure value seems superior in predictive value as compared to the systolic or diastolic values alone. Among patients with a diastolic pressure of 95 mm Hg, for example, a higher pulse pressure simply means that there is a higher systolic pressure which itself is a risk factor for worse outcomes. The pulse pressure also must be considered in the context of the absolute values of systolic and diastolic pressures (e.g., a blood pressure of 120/80 mm Hg is not equivalent in risk to 160/120 mm Hg).

PULSE PRESSURE AND AGE

Both the SBP and DBP are predictive of adverse events from CVD among patients of <55 years age. However, in patients after the age of 55 years, since the DBP declines on average, its predictive value is reduced.

By comparison, the systolic pressure continues to increase with every decade of life, which results in the maintenance of its predictive value for CVD. Thus, in older patients, the association between an increased systolic pressure alone and CVD becomes much stronger than that observed with the DBP alone.

As the age increases, there is a more close correlation between pulse pressure and the systolic pressure as compared with the diastolic pressure. Thus, in the elderly, it is also a good predictor of CVD. An added advantage of the pulse pressure is that it incorporates both the elevation in systolic pressure and the reduction in diastolic pressure, which is noted with age. In some of the cases, this measurement shows superior predictive power than that noted with the systolic pressure alone.

FACTORS RESULTING IN INCREASED PULSE PRESSURE

Elevation in the pulse pressure is a result of factors, which elevate and/or reduce the systolic pressure and diastolic pressure, respectively.
- *Increase in systolic pressure*: This, specifically in the elder individuals, is generally the outcome of stiffness in the large arteries and an early pulse wave reflection. While increased peripheral vascular resistance in younger patients (30–49 years old) seems a relatively more important component of hypertension, the role of peripheral vascular resistance in hypertension decreases gradually with age. Due to the known effects of aging on stiffness

of vessel, elevations in pulse pressure among old age patients (i.e., >55 years age) are caused due to aortic stiffening; whereas, elevations in young age patients (i.e., <45 years age) are more likely to be caused due to increase in stroke volume.
- *Decrease in diastolic pressure*: Since stiffening of the aorta with age reduces the elastic reservoir capacity, more blood runs off from each stroke volume during systole, resulting in a reduced blood volume within the aorta at the onset of diastole. This factor, when combined with diminished elastic recoil and an increased pressure decay rate, causes a fall in the diastolic pressure with age. These changes in diastolic pressure (both in normotensive and hypertensive patients) become evident after the age of 55 years.

Genetics

Increased pulse pressure may be a heritable trait. As an example, a Genome-wide association study that included >120,000 individuals of European ancestry found five loci that were significantly associated with pulse pressure, including three that had opposite effects on systolic and diastolic pressure. One of these five loci, the fidgetin gene, was also associated with pulse pressure in an Asian cohort. Other genetic studies have found a high degree of heritability (ranging from 20 to 40%) with linkage to chromosome 18 in all ethnic groups, chromosome 19 in whites, and chromosome 17 in Hispanics.

Other Considerations

Since a portion of the systolic pressure depends upon the height of the patient, shorter patients tend to have a higher pulse pressure. In addition, slower heart rates result in a greater pulse pressure.

In general, women are shorter than men but tend to have faster heart rates. As a result, differences in pulse pressure with gender are generally lacking since the effect of height on pulse pressure may be counterbalanced by the effect of heart rate.

Increasing evidence suggests that patients with metabolic syndrome have stiffer vessels, resulting in an increased pulse pressure.

Although it is generally thought that the aorta increases in size with age, some studies suggest that increases in pulse pressure are associated with reductions, not increases, in aortic diameter. Data suggest that aortic dimensions may contribute to, rather than result from, increased pulse pressure.

■ INCREASED PULSE PRESSURE AND ADVERSE OUTCOMES

An elevation in the pulse pressure causes more stress on arteries, which leads to fatigue as well as an enhanced fracture rate in the elastic components of the vessel wall. The vascular intima becomes susceptible to damage, thus enhancing the risk of atherosclerosis as well as thrombosis.

- *Pulse pressure and CVD*: In addition to damage to the vascular wall, an increased pulse pressure is associated with increased stress on the left ventricle, which can result in ventricular hypertrophy and failure. Elevated pressure during systole enhances the requirement of myocardial oxygen. For coronary perfusion, the lower diastolic value may act as a limiting factor, which leads to ischemia. The net outcome of these combined effects is that increases in pulse pressure may be a predictor for diverse adverse cardiovascular outcomes.

    The following studies illustrate the range of findings from population-based cohorts:
    - In the Framingham Heart Study, for example, each 10 mm Hg increment in pulse pressure was associated with a 23% higher risk of developing coronary heart disease. This association with pulse pressure was primarily seen in patients over the age of 50 years, particularly over the age of 60 years.
    - In the MRFIT aged 35–57 years without pre-existing diabetes or coronary heart disease, pulse pressure was independently associated with risk, particularly among older men (aged 45–57 years).
    - According to the SHEP trial, which included elderly patients who had isolated systolic hypertension, there was an association of each 10 mm Hg increase in pulse pressure in the active treatment group with elevation in the risk for heart failure by 32% or stroke by 24%, after controlling for systolic pressure as well as other known risk factors.
- *Pulse pressure and diabetes*: Higher pulse pressure was significantly associated with an increased risk of developing diabetes in the CASE-J (Candesartan Antihypertensive Survival Evaluation in Japan) trial.
- *Pulse pressure and progression of chronic kidney disease (CKD)*: Pulse pressure, as a reflection of arterial stiffness, may be an independent risk factor for progression of CKD. In a post-hoc analysis of the RENAAL trial after controlling for multiple potential confounders, a 10 mm Hg higher pulse pressure was significantly associated with a 17% higher relative risk of developing end-stage renal disease. Pulse pressure is also independently associated with urine protein excretion.

PULSE PRESSURE AND ANTIHYPERTENSIVE THERAPY

An analysis of data from clinical trials including >28,000 subjects suggested that the cardiovascular benefit of antihypertensive therapy was mostly linked to SBP control. In addition, the reduction in systolic pressure with treatment was found to be progressively larger than the reduction in DBP with increasing age (e.g., greater fall in pulse pressure with increasing age).

It is premature to use pulse pressure, however, as a factor in deciding which antihypertensive agent to employ or to use the measurement as a treatment endpoint itself. Further prospective research is required to define pulse pressure as a predictor of cardiovascular outcomes, and to determine whether pulse pressure is a better index of response to therapy. The pulse pressure probably best serves as a tool in clinical trials, to better illustrate the pharmacodynamic effects of drugs, and possibly to provide a sharpened estimate of overall CVD risk.

KEY POINTS

- Pulse pressure is defined as the systolic minus the diastolic pressure.
- Increased pulse pressure may be due to either or both an increase in systolic or a decrease in DBP.
- Among older patients, increased systolic pressure results from increased stiffness in the aorta and other large arteries; among younger patients, increased stroke volume plays a more important role.
- Decreased diastolic pressure results from a reduction in aortic blood volume at the onset of diastole. This is related to the age-related decrease in elasticity of the aorta which causes more blood to run off during systole.
- The pulse pressure is a good predictor of cardiovascular events among elderly patients and in some cases, has superior predictive capability to that provided by systolic pressure alone. The best use of pulse pressure is in revising upward the risk estimate provided by the systolic pressure in older individuals.
- Limited data suggest that different hypertensive agents may have varying effects on pulse pressure.

SUGGESTED READING

1. Franklin SS, Gustin W 4th, Wong ND, et al. Hemodynamic patterns of age-related changes in blood pressure. The Framingham Heart Study. Circulation. 1997;96(1):308-15.
2. Winston GJ, Palmas W, Lima J, et al. Pulse pressure and subclinical cardiovascular disease in the multi-ethnic study of atherosclerosis. Am J Hypertens. 2013;26(5):636-42.
3. Franklin SS, Khan SA, Wong ND, et al. Is pulse pressure useful in predicting risk for coronary heart disease? The Framingham heart study. Circulation. 1999;100(4):354-60.
4. Vaccarino V, Berger AK, Abramson J, et al. Pulse pressure and risk of cardiovascular events in the systolic hypertension in the elderly program. Am J Cardiol. 2001;88(9):980-6.

SECTION 3
Interesting ECGs in Hypertension

M Chenniappan

CASE 1: Left Ventricular Hypertrophy

INTRODUCTION
One of the most common ECG changes in hypertension is left ventricular hypertrophy (LVH). There are many ECG criteria for diagnosing LVH in ECG. In this segment, we are highlighting the ECG changes of LVH and its importance in diagnosis and prognosis.

HISTORY

ECG Number 1
This is the ECG of the patient who is a known case of hypertension with a BP of 150/100 mm Hg.

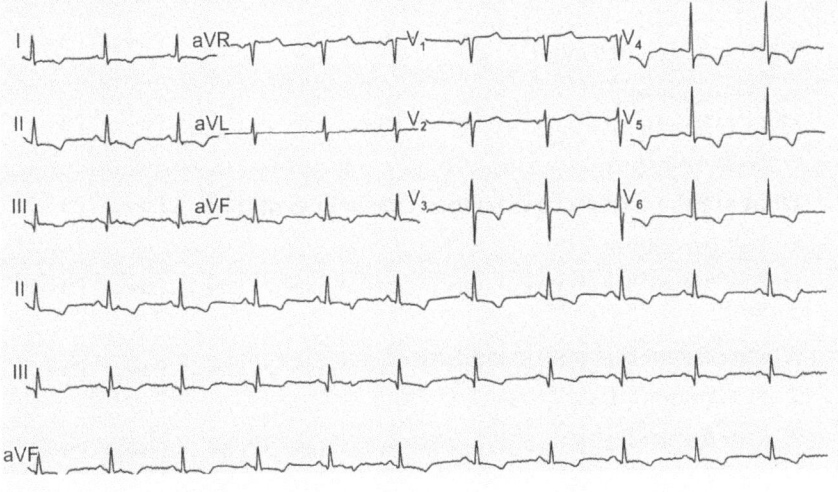

ECG Number 1: 1 mV STD 25 mm/s
ECG courtesy: Dr Venkatesan.

ECG Number 2

This is the ECG of the patient who has similar history and BP as of the patient number 1.

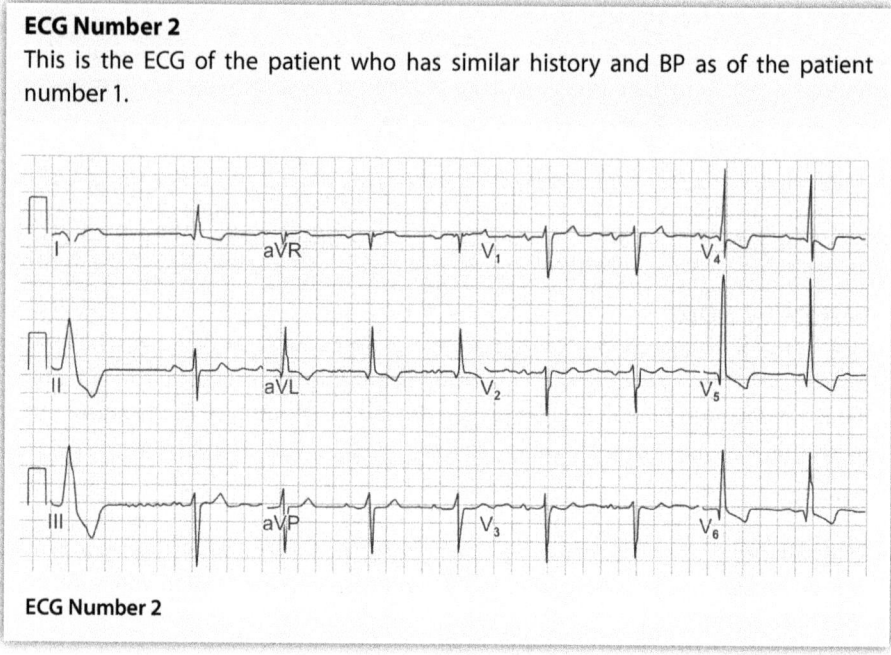

ECG Number 2

Q1. Which patient has LVH?
   a. ECG number 1
   b. ECG number 2
   c. Both a and b

Q2. What are the criteria to diagnose LVH in ECG number 1?
   a. Voltage criteria
   b. Nonvoltage criteria
   c. Both

Q3. Which patient has poor prognosis?
   a. ECG number 1
   b. ECG number 2

Ans. 1-c, 2-b, 3-a

Explanation:
Ans. 3. The patient with the first ECG has low voltage LVH and has poor prognosis.

■ KEY POINTS

- The ECG has high specificity and low sensitivity to detect chamber enlargements which means that if LVH is there in ECG, LVH is definitely present whereas normal ECG does not rule out LVH.

- *LVH*: One of the important target organ diseases (TOD) is LVH. The presence of LVH for the same level of blood pressure (BP) enhances the risk of coronary artery disease (CAD), heart failure, and arrhythmias. Although Echo is ideal to detect LVH, the ECG remains a cost-effective method of detecting LVH.
- *Voltage criteria*:
  - *Limb leads*:
    - R wave in lead I + S wave in lead III >25 mm
    - R wave in aVL >11 mm
    - R wave in aVF >20 mm
    - S wave in aVR >14 mm
  - *Precordial leads*:
    - R wave in V_4, V_5, or V_6 >26 mm
    - R wave in V_5 or V_6 plus S wave in V_1 >35 mm
    - Largest R wave plus largest S wave in precordial leads >45 mm

  Limb lead criteria are used in children and patients with chronic obstructive pulmonary disease (COPD) in whom chest lead criteria may not be reliable.
- *Nonvoltage criteria*:
  - Increased R wave peak time >50 ms in leads V_5 or V_6
  - ST segment depression and T-wave inversion in the left-sided leads: The left ventricular "strain" pattern.

    Voltage criteria must be accompanied by nonvoltage criteria to be considered diagnostic of LVH.
- Usually LVH is diagnosed when high voltage is present. Sometimes the presence of downsloping ST segment with asymmetrical T inversion may be the sole presentation of LVH without high voltage criteria and it is known as "low-voltage LVH".
- *"Low-voltage LVH"*: LVH with interstitial fibrosis may not produce high voltage because of lack of healthy muscle; still it may produce ST-T changes due to abnormal repolarization.
- Diabetic hypertensives and chronic kidney disease (CKD) patients also may not have voltage criteria because of associated fibrosis.
- Obesity, thick chest wall, and COPD also may not have voltage criteria.
- The other ECG signs of fibrosis are widening of QRS, fractured QRS, and pathological Q waves.
- So the take home point is that one should be aware of nonvoltage criteria and look for it in all cases of hypertension which gives the prognosis better than voltage criteria.

CASE 2: Left Bundle Branch Block in Hypertension

INTRODUCTION
Left bundle branch block (LBBB) is most often associated with disease. In hypertension, presence of LBBB will make it difficult to diagnose left ventricular hypertrophy (LVH) in view of altered sequence of depolarization. In this segment, we try to understand the diagnostic difficulties and prognostic implications of LBBB in hypertension.

HISTORY
This is the ECG of the patient who presents with hypertension for further management.

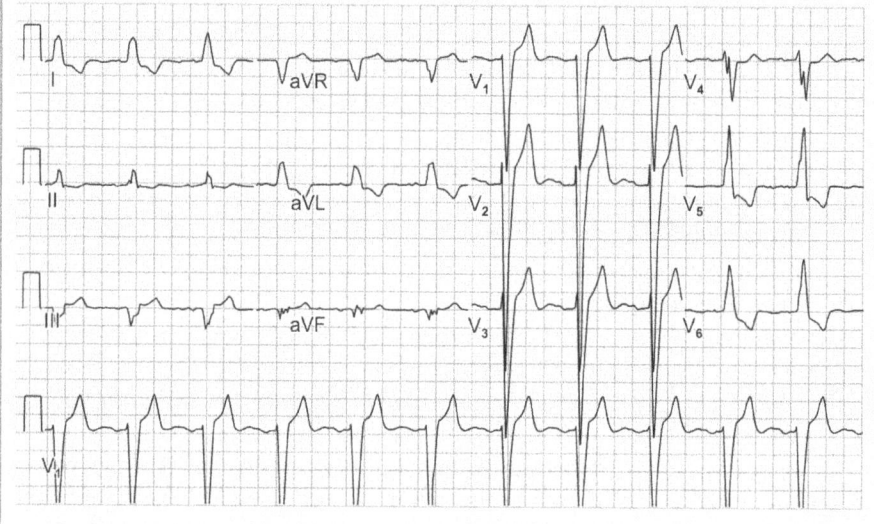

Q1. This ECG shows:
   a. LBBB
   b. LVH
   c. Both

Q2. Does the same voltage criteria to diagnose LVH apply to diagnose LVH in the presence of LBBB?
   a. Yes
   b. No

Q3. What are the prognostic implications?
   a. Bad prognosis
   b. Good prognosis
   c. No prognostic implications

Ans. 1-c, 2-b, 3-a

Explanation:
Ans. 2. No; there is a different voltage criterion to diagnose LVH in the presence of LBBB.
Ans. 3. Bad prognosis; For the same level of BP, the presence of LBBB indicates bad prognosis.

KEY POINTS

- It is always difficult to diagnose LVH in the presence of LBBB and vice versa as LVH can produce QRS widening and LBBB can produce high voltage.
- Various criteria have been proposed and one of them is R in V_5, V_6, and S wave in V_1 is >45 mm (instead of 35 in pure LVH).
- QRS widening >160 ms and LA enlargement are the other supporting criteria.
- LBBB even in the absence of LVH is associated with systolic and diastolic dysfunction and high rate of clinical events.
- In older adults, new onset of LBBB indicates advanced and advancing heart disease.
- In the presence of LBBB and LVH, the presence of LA abnormality and left axis deviation indicates LV dysfunction.
- In uncomplicated LBBB, QRS and ST-T are discordant; if there is concordant QRS and ST-T (QRS and ST-T in the same direction), it may indicate additional CAD.
- In the presence of LBBB, one should always look for additional conduction disturbances such as prolonged PR which may indicate advanced conduction disturbances.
- In the absence of organic disease, existence of LBBB is unusual.
- New LBBB is traditionally believed to be part of the criteria for thrombolysis in the context of chest pain. For avoiding unnecessary thrombolysis, applying Sgarbossa criteria in this situation is always a good practice.

CASE 3: Ventricular Premature Depolarizations in Hypertension

INTRODUCTION
Ventricular premature depolarizations (VPDs) indicate increased irritability of ventricles. In this segment, we try to understand the implications of VPDs in the ECG of a patient with hypertension.

HISTORY
This is the ECG of the patient with hypertension who complains of palpitations.

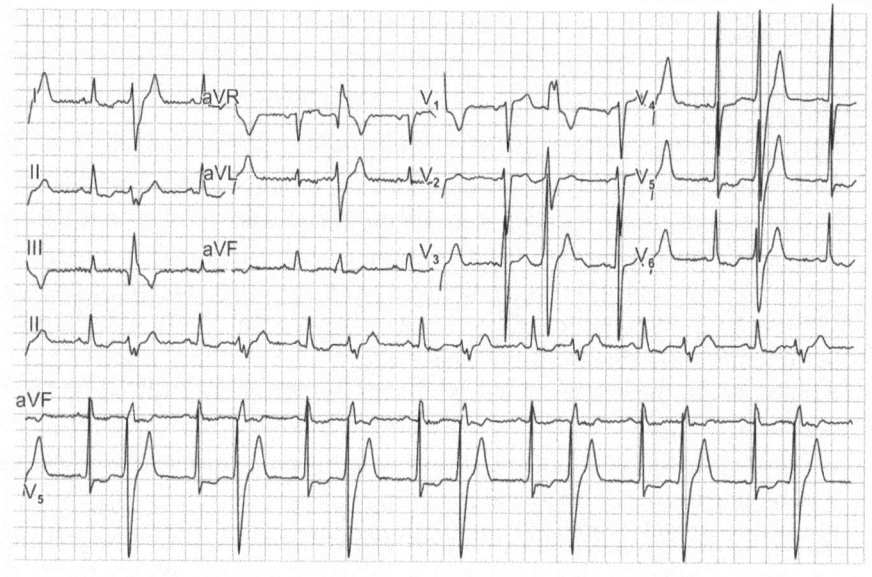

Q1. What is the site of origin of the ventricular premature depolarizations?
   a. Right ventricle
   b. Left ventricle

Q2. Are the ventricular premature depolarizations benign?
   a. Yes
   b. No

Q3. Which drug is preferred in this situation?
   a. Amiodarone
   b. Beta-blockers
   c. Flecainide

Ans. 1-b, 2-b, 3-b

Explanation:
Ans. 2. The VPDs are likely to be malignant because of the following three points:
1. *Frequency:* Bigeminy
2. *Site:* Left ventricle
3. *In the presence of structural heart disease:* LVH

KEY POINTS

- VPDs can occur in hypertension due to various reasons such as left ventricular hypertrophy (LVH), electrolyte disturbances, coronary artery disease (CAD), LV dysfunction, and comorbidities.
- It is crucial to decide whether VPD needs treatment or not.
- It is advisable not to treat all VPDs as many antiarrhythmic drugs such as amiodarone are more dangerous than VPD itself.
- VPDs in the presence of structural heart diseases such as LVH, LV dysfunction, and CAD should be given lot of importance.
- Very frequent VPDs, such as bigeminy, need attention.
- Repetitive VPDs such as couplets and runs can lead on to dangerous ventricular arrhythmias such as VT and ventricular fibrillation.
- Short broad VPDs with notches in upstroke or downstroke are likely to be malignant when compared to tall lean VPDs which are most often benign.
- VPDs with homophasic ST-T changes, i.e., ST-T in the same direction of QRS, may be the subtle sign of associated CAD.
- If VPD is positive in V_1, it is likely from LV and if VPD is predominantly negative in V_1, it is likely from RV. Most often, RVOT VPDs are benign.
- It must be remembered that beta-blockers are safe and effective anti-arrhythmic drugs.

CASE 4: Beyond Left Ventricular Hypertrophy

INTRODUCTION
Although we always look for left ventricular hypertrophy (LVH) in the ECG of the patient, there are other signs in the ECG which may be of importance. In this segment, we look at one such important finding.

HISTORY
This is the ECG of the patient with hypertension who complains of dyspnea.

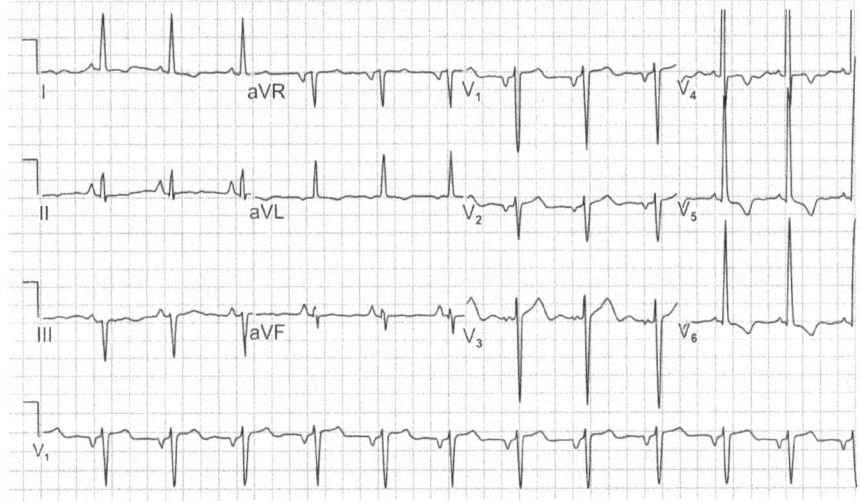

Q1. This ECG shows the cause of dyspnea:
   a. Yes
   b. No

Q2. This ECG shows only LVH:
   a. Yes
   b. No

Q3. This ECG shows LV dysfunction:
   a. Yes
   b. No

Ans. 1-a, 2-b, 3-a

Explanation:

Ans. 3. In addition to LVH, the ECG shows deep terminal negative component of P in V_1 which is suggestive of raised LA pressures and LV dysfunction.

■ KEY POINTS

- In all patients with hypertension, one should always look at P wave in V_1.
- The deep terminal negative component of P in V_1 which is >0.04 seconds in width and >1 square in depth is suggestive of LA abnormality even in the absence of LVH.
- This abnormality of P wave is suggestive of raised LA pressure even in the absence of other criteria of LA enlargement.
- P wave terminal force (PWTF) was calculated by measuring the duration of P wave in seconds multiplied by the P wave amplitude of the negative terminal portion of the P wave in V_1 in millimeters.
- Then patients were categorized into two groups. In the first group, PWTF was >-0.04 mm/s (smaller than one small square). In the second group, the PWTF was ≤-0.04 mm/s (larger than one small square).
- The second group of patients who have P terminal force larger than one small box is likely to develop complications like AF and stroke.
- This may also indicate LV dysfunction systolic, diastolic or both.
- In serial ECGs, progressive deepening of P in V_1 is suggestive of ongoing LV dysfunction.
- In hypertensive patients presenting with dyspnea and preserved LV ejection fraction, the deep negative component of P in V_1 is suggestive of heart failure with preserved ejection fraction (HFpEF).
- Of all ECG signs, the P wave depth in V_1 has the highest hazard ratio for cardiovascular death.

CASE 5: The T Wave in Hypertension

INTRODUCTION
In hypertension, ECG not only shows target organ diseases like left ventricular hypertrophy (LVH) and LV dysfunction, but also shows clues regarding complications of hypertension. In this segment, we look at one such complication which mimics the other complications.

HISTORY
This is the ECG of a patient with hypertension who comes with disturbance in consciousness.

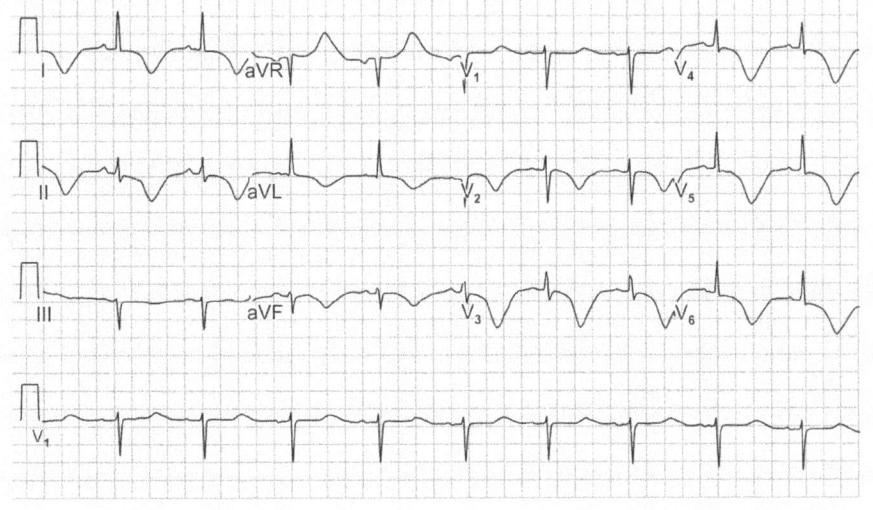

Q1. This ECG shows acute coronary syndrome (ACS):
   a. Yes
   b. No

Q2. This ECG shows electrolyte disturbance:
   a. Yes
   b. No

Q3. This ECG is suggestive of cerebrovascular accident:
   a. Yes
   b. No

Ans. 1-b, 2-b, 3-a
Explanation:
Ans. 3. The T-wave inversion is deep broad and splayed with prolonged QT interval which is suggestive of cerebrovascular accident.

KEY POINTS

- The T wave in hypertension gives lot of clues regarding the etiology, complications, and drug and electrolyte effects in hypertension.
- In CVA, a complication of hypertension, the T-wave inversion can be broad and splayed with QT prolongation.
- If the T-wave inversion is symmetrical and deep with normal QT, it is suggestive of coronary artery disease (CAD) (Complication).
- If T-wave inversion is asymmetrical and associated with downsloping ST-segment, it is secondary ST-T change due to LVH (Target organ disease).
- If the T wave is tall with narrow base and sharp apex, it is due to hyperkalemia which may indicate secondary cause of hypertension due to chronic kidney disease (Etiology).
- Hyperkalemia may be also due to angiotensin inhibitors and aldosterone antagonists (Drug effects).
- The tall T with broad base and blunt apex is due to subendocardial ischemia which presents as ACS (Complication).
- The low voltage T with prominent U is suggestive of hypokalemia which may indicate primary hyperaldosteronism as the cause of hypertension (Etiology).
- Hypokalemic ECG changes can also occur due to diuretic therapy with thiazide and loop diuretics (Drug effect).
- The tall T waves with prolonged ST segment usually occur in CKD due to hypocalcemia which prolongs ST segment and hyperkalemia which produces tall T wave (Etiology).

SECTION 4
Issues in Diagnosis

Nihar P Mehta

CASE 1: Role of Home Blood Pressure Monitoring in Patients with Hypertension

A 45-year-old male is a known case of diabetes, hypertension, and chronic kidney disease presented to the physician with intermittent headaches. He has no addictions and is compliant with his medication. He is currently on tablet metformin 500 mg three times a day, olmesartan 40 mg once a day, and amlodipine 5 mg twice a day.

The following are his vital signs during his clinical visit:
- Afebrile
- BMI: 28 kg/m^2
- Heart rate: 78 beats/min
- Blood pressure: 144/94 mm Hg in the right arm in sitting position.

The following are the patient's blood reports:
- Hemoglobin: 11.2 g/dL
- Total leukocyte count: 6,700/μL
- Platelet count: 344,000/μL
- Fasting blood sugar: 104 mg/dL
- Postprandial blood sugar: 133 mg/dL
- HbA1c: 6.4%
- Creatinine: 1.8 mg/dL
- Sodium: 137 mmol/L
- Potassium: 4.7 mmol/L
- Chloride: 100 mmol/L

The physician advised him to continue his medications and to start home blood pressure monitoring (HBPM).

Q1. When should the physician advise the patient to follow-up with his HBPM?
   a. 3 days
   b. 5 days
   c. 7 days
   d. 14 days
   e. 30 days

Q2. While advising the patient about the method of home BP measurement, which of the following statements of the physician is true?
   a. The patient should lie down on a flat surface for 5 minutes before taking the BP reading
   b. The readings should be taken randomly at any time of the day
   c. Home BP is defined as the average of 10 consecutive BP readings
   d. Regular activities like bathing, drinking coffee or exercise do not interfere with the HBPM readings
   e. Each time, two readings should be taken separated by 1–2 minutes

Q3. During follow-up of the HBPM readings, which of the following HBPM readings is most significant for the physician to monitor and adjust the patient's treatment?
   a. A single reading of 160/100 mm Hg
   b. More than 50% of reading >140 mm Hg systolic and 90 mm Hg diastolic
   c. Average of 12 readings >135 mm Hg systolic and 85 mm Hg diastolic
   d. Average of 12 readings >125 mm Hg systolic and 75 mm Hg diastolic
   e. Three consecutive readings >140 mm Hg systolic and 90 mm Hg diastolic

Q4. Which of the following associated conditions would be a deterrent for the physician to advise HBPM for this patient?
   a. Associated microalbuminuria
   b. Associated atrial fibrillation
   c. Past history of heart failure with a normal ejection fraction
   d. During pregnancy
   e. Past history of cerebrovascular accident

Q5. All of the following statements about HBPM are true except:
   a. HBPM devices are oscillometric devices
   b. Wrist monitors are as accurate as brachial (arm) monitors
   c. The devices should be calibrated against mercury sphygmomanometers every 6–12 months
   d. HBPM is more predictive of adverse outcomes [e.g., stroke, end-stage renal disease (ESRD)] than clinic blood pressure monitoring
   e. The cuff width should equal to 40% of the mid arm circumference and the cuff length should equal to 80% of the mid arm circumference

Ans. 1-c, 2-e, 3-c, 4-b, 5-b

■ EXPLANATIONS

Answers 1 and 2

Method of home blood pressure monitoring:
- Patient should sit calmly with the back support, feet flat on floor for 5 minutes before taking a reading. The legs should not be crossed.
- Caffeine, smoking, alcohol, bathing, and exercise should be avoided for at least 30 minutes before the reading is taken.

- The upper arm should be bare.
- When taking a reading, the arm should be supported on a firm surface (table or armrest) at heart level.
- The cuff should fit snugly on the arm, about ½-1 inch above the elbow crease.

Schedule of BP readings:
- Readings should be routinely taken in the morning before medication and at night before bed.
- Each time, patients should take at least two readings separated by 1-2 minutes between readings (four readings each day).
- Readings should be taken twice every day for 7 consecutive days.
- Readings of the first day to be discarded.
- This gives a total of at least 12 readings. Home BP is defined as the average of these readings.
- In patients with stable BP, this process of 12-14 measurements over 1 week should be repeated every 3 months to ensure adequate BP control.
- Proper documentation of the date, time, and blood pressure readings is essential.

Answer 3
Interpretation of HBPM
- The upper limit of normal for home BP is 135/85 mm Hg.
- This corresponds to a clinic BP of 140/90 mm Hg.

Threshold levels of BP for diagnosis of hypertension:

	SBP (mm Hg)	DBP (mm Hg)
Office	≥140	≥90
Home BP monitoring	>135	>85
Ambulatory BP monitoring day	>140	>90
Ambulatory BP monitoring night	>125	>75
Ambulatory 24-hour BP monitoring	>135	>85

(SBP: systolic blood pressure; DBP: diastolic blood pressure)

- Patient should be educated to understand the readings.
- A single increased BP value does not warrant an immediate alarm. In such cases, BP of the patient should be recorded many more times and the concerned physician should be consulted. Only if the blood pressure reaches a systolic >180 mm Hg or diastolic >110 mm Hg, he/she should immediately alert the physician.

Answer 4
Contraindications for HBPM
Home monitoring devices for measuring blood pressure use oscillometric methods which may not provide exact values for patients suffering from atrial fibrillation or other arrhythmias.

Recommendations for Use of HBPM[1]

- The use of HBPM is indicated in the cases of patients with suspected or newly diagnosed hypertension, where it may differentiate between white-coat and sustained hypertension. If the values are ambiguous, ambulatory BP monitoring becomes essential to confirm the diagnosis.
- Masked hypertension may be diagnosed in patients with prehypertension with the help of HBPM.
- HBPM is recommended to assess the reaction or effect of the antihypertensive treatment prescribed and may improve adherence.
- HBPM helps elderly patients in whom both BP variability and the white-coat effects are elevated.
- Diabetic patients can use HBPM as a valuable option as they require strict control of BP.
- HBPM may be a suitable choice for pregnant women, children, and patients with kidney disease.

Answer 5

Equipment for HBPM

- Fully automated monitors that use the brachial artery (arm) for measurements are the most reliable.
- Wrist monitors are not recommended.
- Oscillometric devices may not work well with patients who have atrial fibrillation or other arrhythmias.
- Patients monitor should be calibrated against mercury sphygmomanometer every 6–12 months.
- A regular adult size cuff may not be appropriate for everyone. The cuff size actually refers to the size of the bladder inside. The cuff width should equal 40% of the mid arm circumference and the cuff length should equal to 80% of the mid arm circumference.
- If cuff used is too small, it causes overestimation of BP. If cuff used is too wide, it causes underestimation of BP.
- HBPM correlates more closely with the results of ambulatory BP monitoring than clinic BP readings; hence HBPM is more predictive of adverse outcomes (e.g., stroke, ESRD) than clinic BP.[2]

CASE 2: Role of Ambulatory Blood Pressure Monitoring in Patients with Hypertension

INTRODUCTION
The diagnosis and management of a hypertensive patient is more than the simple measurement of the blood pressure with a sphygmomanometer. Often patients seemingly well-controlled develop end-organ damage and some patients, on the other hand, have large fluctuations of blood pressure. Some of the most challenging cases are those who do not achieve blood pressure control in spite of several antihypertensive medications in maximal doses. It is important to diagnose the subset of hypertensive patients with masked hypertension, white coat hypertension, resistant hypertension, and labile hypertension. The following case scenarios describe the typical presentation of different challenging subsets of hypertensive patients.

Five patients presented to the hypertension clinic with different presentation. They all fall into specific different categories of hypertension among the following:
a. Masked hypertension
b. White coat hypertension
c. Pseudo hypertension
d. Resistant hypertension
e. Labile hypertension

MASKED HYPERTENSION
Patient 1
A 48-year-old male underwent investigations for intermittent headaches. His ECG showed left ventricular hypertrophy. His echocardiography showed ejection fraction of 65% with concentric left ventricular hypertrophy. His office BP was measured on three separate occasions and the readings were as follows: 136/88 mm Hg, 134/84 mm Hg, and 138/88 mm Hg.

He was advised home BP monitoring which showed average reading of 148/96 mm Hg.

Which of the above categories of hypertension would he fall into?

WHITE COAT HYPERTENSION
Patient 2
A 48-year-old male is a known case of hypertension on amlodipine 5 mg twice a day and telmisartan 40 mg twice a day. His ECG and 2D echocardiography are normal and there is no evidence of end organ damage on other investigations.

His clinic BP was measured on three separate occasions, which showed the following readings: 144/90 mm Hg, 150/88 mm Hg, and 148/92 mm Hg.

He was advised home BP monitoring which showed average reading of 130/80 mm Hg.

Which of the above categories of hypertension would he fall into?

PSEUDO HYPERTENSION
Patient 3
A 78-year-old hypertensive patient with chronic kidney disease and on hemodialysis presented to the clinic for a regular follow-up. He was taking amlodipine 5 mg twice a day, nebivolol 5 mg once a day, and prazosin 2.5 mg once a day for controlling his BP.

His clinic BP readings on 3 separate days, when taken with a mercury sphygmomanometer, were as follows: 150/90 mm Hg, 154/96 mm Hg, and 160/94 mm Hg.

His clinic BP readings, when taken on the same days, with an automated oscillometric device, were as follows: 138/80 mm Hg, 140/84 mm Hg, and 144/80 mm Hg.

Which of the above categories of hypertension would he fall into?

RESISTANT HYPERTENSION
Patient 4
A 54-year-old obese female patient with chronic hypertension, T2DM, and dyslipidemia presented to the clinic 2 months ago with uncontrolled hypertension. Her medications were increased to the following:
- Tablet telmisartan 40 mg twice a day.
- Tablet hydrochlorothiazide 25 mg twice a day.
- Tablet cilnidipine 10 mg once a day.
- Tablet metoprolol 50 mg twice a day.

During her current visit, her clinic BP was 134/86 mm Hg.

Her average home BP measurement was 128/82 mm Hg.

Which of the above categories of hypertension would she fall into?

LABILE HYPERTENSION
Patient 5
A 32-year-old female with recurrent episodes of headaches, sweating, and palpitations was found to have a blood pressure of 160/102 mm Hg by a physician. At the hypertension clinic, her BP was found to be 128/78 mm Hg.

She was advised home BP monitoring and her readings of the first 3 days were as follows:

	Morning BP (mm Hg)	Evening BP (mm Hg)
Day 1	124/78	154/94
Day 2	174/102	128/76
Day 3	132/80	184/110

Which of the above categories of hypertension would she fall into?

Ans. 1-b, 2-a, 3-d, 4-e, 5-c

EXPLANATIONS

Patient 1: Masked Hypertension or Isolated Ambulatory Hypertension

Patients who are normotensive by clinic/office BP measurements but are hypertensive by ambulatory BP monitoring or home BP monitoring are referred to as "masked hypertension" cases. It can be seen in as many as 10–40% of patients who are normotensive by clinic BP measurement. Patients in whom the BP values are normal clinically but have the evidence of end organ damage of hypertension such as hypertensive retinopathy, microalbuminuria, and left ventricular hypertrophy are suspected to have masked hypertension. Such patients are at an increased risk of sustained hypertension and cardiovascular morbidity.

Patient 2: White Coat Hypertension or Isolated Clinic/Office Hypertension

Patients with average clinic BP reading >140/90 mm Hg and ambulatory BP monitoring or home BP monitoring readings averagely in the normotensive range are referred to as "white coat hypertension" cases.

The white coat effect occurs due to anxiety while visiting the physician. The prevalence of white coat hypertension is in the range of 10–20%. The white coat effect is seen more often in children and elderly. The white coat effect also reduces when an assistant, technician or nurse, rather than the physician, does BP measurement. Automated oscillometric BP monitors also reduce the white coat effect.

The cardiovascular risk associated with white coat hypertension is slightly higher when compared to normotensive patients however, it is much lower than the risk associated with sustained hypertension or masked hypertension. Patients with white coat hypertension do stand a higher risk of development of sustained hypertension and careful monitoring is warranted.

Patient 3: Pseudohypertension

In patients who have stiff vessels due to marked arterial calcification, compression of the brachial artery may require a cuff pressure higher than the actual systolic pressure. This leads to systolic and diastolic pressures being higher by 10 mm Hg or more when measured by a mercury sphygmomanometer as compared to the BP measured using oscillometric devices or direct intra-arterial blood pressure. This phenomenon is called pseudohypertension.

Cuff-inflation Hypertension

While self-measuring BP using a sphygmomanometer, the muscular activity used to inflate the cuff can cause an acute elevation of blood pressure. This is called cuff-inflation hypertension. This effect usually reduces within 5–20 seconds. Thus, when self-measuring BP, the cuff should be inflated to about 30 mm Hg above the estimated systolic BP and the fall in the pressure should be no >2–3 mm Hg/s. This would allow the effect of the muscular activity to dissipate. This problem can be avoided by using automated oscillometric devices.

Patient 4: Resistant Hypertension

It is defined as a clinical condition in which the blood pressure remains above the target levels despite the use of three antihypertensive drugs belonging to different classes (one of them being a diuretic). Patients in whom the target BP levels are achieved with four or more antihypertensive drugs also fall under the category of resistant hypertension.

Refractory Hypertension

It is defined as a clinical condition in which the blood pressure levels cannot be controlled despite using the maximum tolerated doses of five or more antihypertensive drugs (two of them being chlorthalidone and a mineralocorticoid receptor antagonist), under the care of a hypertensive specialist.

Patient 5: Labile Hypertension

Labile hypertension is characterized by sudden abrupt fluctuation in the BP, varying from normal BP to hypertension at different times of the day.

Causes of labile hypertension can be a pheochromocytoma, emotional factors like fear or anxiety, panic attacks, white coat hypertension, excessive salt intake or excessive caffeine intake, anesthesia, etc.

REFERENCES

1. Pickering TG, Miller NH, Ogedegbe G, et al. Call to action on use and reimbursement for home blood pressure monitoring: executive summary: a joint scientific statement from the American Heart Association, American Society Of Hypertension, and Preventive Cardiovascular Nurses Association. Hypertens Dallas Tex 1979. 2008;52(1):1-9.
2. Niiranen TJ, Hänninen M-R, Johansson J, et al. Home-measured blood pressure is a stronger predictor of cardiovascular risk than office blood pressure: The Finn-Home study. Hypertension. 2010;55(6):1346-51.

SECTION 5
Hypertension in Pregnancy

Falguni S Parikh

CASE 1: Pregnancy in Aortoarteritis

A 22-year-old primigravida reported for first antenatal checkup with 8 months of amenorrhea and no medical complaints till date. Physical examination revealed absence of upper limb pulses. Only lower limb pulses were palpable and blood pressure could also be recorded in lower limbs only (BP: 90/70 mm Hg). Jugular venous distension was absent. On auscultation, there were normal first and second heart sounds with no murmur.

Significantly high levels of C-reactive protein and ESR (100 mm/h) were seen in initial laboratory investigations while complete blood count, liver and renal function tests, urine analysis, chest X-ray, and fundoscopy results were normal. Electrocardiography revealed normal sinus rhythm. Normal growth of the fetus was revealed by the fetal ultrasound with Doppler velocimetry and no uteroplacental insufficiency was reported.

Keeping a possibility of aortoarteritis, magnetic resonance angiography was done which confirmed narrowing of supra-aortic vessels with normal renal arteries and abdominal aorta.

Q1. **All of the following are diagnostic for Takayasu arteritis (TA) except:**
   a. Age <40 years
   b. BP difference >10 mm Hg
   c. Digital ischemia
   d. Bruit over the arteries
   e. Arteriogram abnormalities

Q2. **Which of the following arteries is not involved in aortoarteritis?**
   a. Pulmonary artery
   b. Renal artery
   c. Subclavian artery
   d. Carotids
   e. All of the above

Q3. **Hypertension in aortoarteritis is contributed due to:**
   a. Renal artery stenosis
   b. Acquired coarctation
   c. Reduced baroreceptor reactivity
   d. Decreased aortic capacitance
   e. All of the above

Q4. Which of the following statement is false?
   a. Steroids are the mainstay of treatment
   b. Cytotoxic drugs can be used in pregnancy
   c. Pregnancy does not appear to exacerbate the disease
   d. Induction of labor is considered in presence of superimposed hypertension
   e. Elective cesarean section is indicated for severe disease

Q5. Most common type of Takayasu among Indians is:
   a. Type I
   b. Type II
   c. Type III
   d. Type IV
   e. Type V

Ans. 1-c, 2-e, 3-e, 4-b, 5-c

DISCUSSION

Takayasu's arteritis is a chronic inflammatory vasculitis that involves the aorta and its major branches. It is also known as aortic arch syndrome, panaortitis, aortitis syndrome, pulseless disease, atypical coarctation of aorta, middle aortic syndrome, Martorell syndrome, occlusive thromboaortopathy, and young female arteritis. The most common vessels involved apart from the aorta are the subclavian artery, renal artery, and common carotid artery.

Takayasu's arteritis is not unfamiliar to any region of the globe but has a prevalence and clinical pattern that differs widely between regions. Japan, India, and South America have a higher prevalence.

It was classified into three types by Ueno et al. in 1967:
- *Type I*: Inflammation is localized to the arch of aorta and its branches.
- *Type II*: Involvement of thoracoabdominal aorta and its branches with no involvement of the arch.
- *Type III*: Combined features of both Type I and Type II.
- *Type IV*: Recommended by Lupi Harrera et al. in 1975. This type shows the features of all the three types along with pulmonary involvement.
- *Type V*: Another variant proposed by Panja et al. that involves the coronary arteries.

The occurrence of the different types is not consistent globally. Agarwal et al. reported the occurrence of these types in India as: Type I (22%), Type II (25%), Type III (53%), and Type IV (26%).

The diagnostic criteria put forth by the American Society of Rheumatology in 1990 for confirming TA are as follows:
- Onset of disease by ≤40 years of age.
- Claudication of extremities

- Decreased pulse rate in brachial artery.
- Difference of >10 mm Hg in systolic blood pressure (SBP) as recorded between both the arms.
- Bruit over subclavian artery or aorta
- Abnormal aortogram

The diagnosis is confirmed if at least "3" of the "6" criteria mentioned above are present. The criteria have a sensitivity and specificity of 90.5% and 97.8%, respectively.

Management of Takayasu's Arteritis
- *Medical therapy*: Steroids and immunosuppressants
- Surgical revascularization
- Balloon angioplasty with or without stents.

Pregnancy and Takayasu's Arteritis

Fertility is not affected by TA and often the disease is encountered in young females during pregnancy. The course of disease seems to be unaffected or worsened by pregnancy.

Features of vascular ischemia or inflammation [such as vascular pain (carotidynia), claudication, diminished or absent pulse, bruit, asymmetric blood pressure in either upper or lower limbs (or both)].

Predominant manifestations arise from effects of uncontrolled hypertension on cardiovascular and renal function along with central nervous system (CNS) and eyes.

Accelerated and uncontrolled hypertension can lead to:
- Pre-eclampsia
- CHF
- Renal failure
- Antepartum hemorrhage

Intracerebral hemorrhage has been described during labor (SBP increase of 20–75 mm Hg during 2nd stage of labor).

High incidence of intrauterine growth restriction: This results due to uncontrolled blood pressure and heart failure.

Poor control of BP, delay in seeking medical treatment, and abdominal aorta involvement are associated with poor fetal outcome.

Steroids are safe during pregnancy.

Timely and appropriate BP control leads to a favorable pregnancy outcome most of the time.

Second stage of labor is cut short during vaginal delivery and C-section is carried out in case of severe disease.

CASE 2: Pre-eclampsia

A 34-year-old lady who was 32 weeks pregnant came for antenatal check-up. She was found to have blood pressure of 170/106 mm Hg and had 1+ proteinuria on urine dipstick testing.

Q1. Other features of severe pre-eclampsia besides blood pressure above 160/110 mm Hg are:
   a. Pulmonary edema
   b. Renal failure
   c. Hepatocellular injury
   d. Thrombocytopenia or coagulopathy
   e. All of the above

Q2. Treatment of pre-eclampsia requires the following except:
   a. Antihypertensive therapy
   b. IV magnesium sulfate for seizure prophylaxis
   c. Bed rest
   d. Aspirin
   e. Frequent blood pressure monitoring

Q3. Which is not a risk factor for pre-eclampsia?
   a. Molar pregnancy
   b. Multigravida
   c. Age >40 years
   d. Multiple pregnancy
   e. Family history

Q4. Hypertension due to pre-eclampsia is largely due to:
   a. Increase in systemic vascular resistance
   b. Decrease in blood volume
   c. Decrease in systemic vascular resistance
   d. Decreased vascular permeability
   e. Increase in blood volume

Q5. Pre-eclampsia can be cured by:
   a. Antihypertensives
   b. Diet alone
   c. Diuretics
   d. Decreased fluid intake
   e. Delivery of the baby

Ans. 1-e, 2-d, 3-b, 4-a, 5-e

DISCUSSION

Hypertension (elevated blood pressure value) during pregnancy can be attributed to four reasons:
1. Pre-eclampsia
2. Chronic hypertension
3. Pre-eclampsia superimposed upon chronic hypertension
4. Gestational hypertension (also called transient hypertension)

Pre-eclampsia is the occurrence of hypertension after 20 weeks of gestation. Pregnant women with pre-eclampsia may be highly susceptible to cardiovascular pathologies in future.

Criteria for the Diagnosis of Pre-eclampsia

Systolic blood pressure ≥140 mm Hg or diastolic blood pressure ≥90 mm Hg on two separate instances with a minimum of 4 hours gap in between after 20 weeks of gestation in a patient with earlier normal blood pressure readings
- In case SBP is ≥160 mm Hg or DBP is ≥110 mm Hg, the condition is established within minutes

and
- Proteinuria ≥0.3 g in a 24-hour urine specimen or protein/creatinine ratio ≥0.3 (mg/mg) (30 mg/mmol)
- Dipstick ≥1+ in case quantitative measurement is not feasible

or
New-onset hypertension with the establishment of at least one of the following criteria (with or without proteinuria):
- Platelet count <100,000/μL
- Serum creatinine >1.1 mg/dL (97.2 μL/L)
- Liver transaminases at least twice the upper limit of the normal concentrations for the local laboratory.
- Pulmonary edema
- Cerebral or visual symptoms (e.g., new-onset and constant headache that do not subside with usual analgesic dose, blurred vision, flashing lights or sparks, scotomata, etc.)

Classification of Pre-eclampsia Based on Degree of Hypertension

Degree of hypertension	Mild (140/90 mm Hg to 149/99 mm Hg)	Moderate (150/100 mm Hg to 159/109 mm Hg)	Severe (160/110 mm Hg or higher)

Risk Factors for Pre-eclampsia
- Hypertension during an earlier pregnancy
- Chronic kidney disease

- Autoimmune diseases such as systemic lupus erythematosus and antiphospholipid syndrome
- Type 1 or type 2 diabetes mellitus
- Chronic hypertension

Women with any of the risk factors mentioned below are classified as being at moderate risk of pre-eclampsia:
- Primigravida
- 40 years of age and above
- An interval of 10 years between pregnancies
- Body mass index (BMI) of 35 kg/m² or more at first check-up
- Familial occurrence of pre-eclampsia
- Multiple pregnancy

Pre-eclampsia with Severe Features of Disease

New onset high blood pressure and proteinuria, in addition to at least one of the following:
- Blurred vision, scotomata, altered mental status, severe headache
- Right upper quadrant or epigastric pain, nausea, vomiting
- Liver enzymes at twice normal levels.
- *Very high BP:* SBP ≥160 mm Hg or DBP ≥110 mm Hg on two separate instances with a gap of minimum 6 hours in between.
- Platelets count <100,000
- Severe proteinuria
- Reduced urine output (<500 mL in 24 hours)
- Restricted fetal growth
- Fluid in the lungs (pulmonary edema) or bluish discoloration of the skin (called cyanosis)
- Stroke

Fetal Effects

- Abnormal nonstress test or biophysical profile score
- Ultrasound reveals retarded fetal growth and reduced amount of amniotic fluid around the fetus.
- Doppler tests reveal reduced umbilical cord blood flow.

The only treatment for pre-eclampsia is delivery of the baby and placenta. Reduced physical activity, but not strict bed rest, and intake of high dosages of blood pressure medication can decrease the blood pressure but will not stop pre-eclampsia from worsening or decrease the risk of its complications.

Anticonvulsant therapy becomes essential as many women with pre-eclampsia can develop seizures (eclampsia). Most frequently prescribed anticonvulsant drug is magnesium sulfate as it not only avoids seizures. It is safe for both mother and baby. The drug is administered intravenously to the pregnant woman during labor and mostly for 24 hours following delivery.

Increased blood pressure and urinary protein resolve post-delivery, within a few days in most cases. Nevertheless, in few cases, the mother may need appropriate drugs to mitigate elevated blood pressure after discharge from the clinic.

CASE 3: Chronic Hypertension in Pregnancy

A 36-year-old lady, 14 weeks pregnant, was referred by gynecologist as she had blood pressure of 160/100 mm Hg. She was diagnosed to have high blood pressure prior to pregnancy a year ago during health check-up, however, had chosen not to take any treatment.

Q1. **What is the likely diagnosis?**
   a. Pregnancy-induced hypertension
   b. Pre-eclampsia
   c. Chronic hypertension
   d. Gestational hypertension
   e. Difficult to say

Q2. **All of the following drugs can be used in pregnancy except:**
   a. Alpha methyldopa
   b. Enalapril
   c. Labetalol
   d. Nifedipine
   e. All of the above

Q3. **What are the causes of pre-existing hypertension in pregnancy?**
   a. Polycystic disease
   b. Pheochromocytoma
   c. Cushing's disease
   d. Renal disease
   e. All of the above

Q4. **In chronic hypertension of pregnancy:**
   a. The perinatal risk is only increased in the presence of proteinuria
   b. The use of thiazide diuretics is associated with teratogenesis
   c. First trimester use of angiotensin-converting enzyme (ACE) inhibitors is an indication for a termination of pregnancy
   d. Methyldopa is free of side effects
   e. The relative risk of pre-eclampsia supervening is more than doubled

Q5. **At what level of blood pressure should the treatment be initiated?**
   a. >160/90 mm Hg
   b. >140/80 mm Hg
   c. >150/90 mm Hg
   d. >130/80 mm Hg
   e. >120/80 mm Hg

Ans. 1-c, 2-b, 3-e, 4-e, 5-a

DISCUSSION

Chronic hypertension in pregnancy is described as the systolic and diastolic blood pressure of not <140 mm Hg and 90 mm Hg, respectively, prior to pregnancy or in those who seek initial clinical care for pregnancy, before 20 weeks of gestation. Eliminating secondary causes of hypertension is very crucial in such cases.

Most women with chronic hypertension have good pregnancy outcomes, but such women are more prone to have pregnancy complications, than the general pregnant population. The more severe the hypertension and end-organ damage, the more is the risk of an adverse outcome.

Chronic hypertensive women have an increased frequency of pre-eclampsia (17–25%; while the figure is as low as 3–5% in the general population), fetal growth restriction, preterm birth, placental abruption, and cesarean section. Prolonged hypertension elevates the risk of superimposed pre-eclampsia.

Most women with chronic hypertension have a reduction in blood pressure during pregnancy, similar to that observed in normotensive women. There is a decrease in BP toward the end of first trimester while the values increase toward pre-pregnancy values during the third trimester. This shows that antihypertensive drugs may be tapered during pregnancy.

With the fact that pre-eclampsia develops in a group of chronic hypertensive women, about 7–20% of women exhibit aggravation of hypertension during pregnancy without the development of pre-eclampsia.

Antihypertensive treatment should be decided accordingly in women with chronic hypertension in childbearing age group, if they are planning pregnancy.

The goal should be to maintain the blood pressure <160/90 mm Hg in pregnant women with uncomplicated chronic hypertension.

Angiotensin-converting enzyme inhibitors and angiotensin II receptor blockers (ARBs) are commonly used antihypertensive medications, but their use should be avoided in pregnant women to avoid susceptibility to congenital abnormalities and thus the pregnant women who use these drugs should use safer agents.

Common Pharmacologic Therapies for Chronic Hypertension in Pregnancy

Drug	Class or mechanism of action	Usual range of dose	Comments
Methyldopa	Centrally acting alpha agonist	250 mg to 1.5 g orally twice daily	• Often used as first-line therapy • Long-term data suggest safety in offspring

Continued

Continued

Drug	Class or mechanism of action	Usual range of dose	Comments
Labetalol	Combined alpha- and beta-blocker	100–1,200 mg orally twice daily	• Often used as first-line therapy • May exacerbate asthma • Intravenous formulation is available to treat hypertensive emergencies
Metoprolol	Beta-blocker	25–200 mg orally twice daily	• May exacerbate asthma • Possible association with fetal growth restriction • Other beta-blockers (e.g., pindolol and propranolol) have been safely used • Some experts recommend avoiding atenolol
Nifedipine (long-acting)	Calcium-channel blocker	30–120 mg orally once daily	• Use of short-acting nifedipine is typically not recommended, given risk of hypotension • Other calcium-channel blockers have been safely used
Hydralazine	Peripheral vasodilator	50–300 mg orally in two or four divided doses	Intravenous formulation is available to treat hypertensive emergencies
Hydrochlorothiazide	Diuretic	12.5–50 mg orally once daily	Previous concerns about increased risk of an adverse outcome are not supported by recent data

> **CASE 4: Eclampsia**
>
> A 24-year-old female primigravida with 36 weeks of gestation was brought to the emergency department with one episode of seizure and altered mentation. She had no previous medical issues and was regularly visiting for antenatal check-ups.
>
> On examination, her blood pressure was 180/100 mm Hg, she was altered and frothing at the mouth, and other systems were normal.

Q1. Indications for IV magnesium sulfate are the following except:
   a. Woman with severe hypertension or severe pre-eclampsia has an eclamptic seizure
   b. Woman with severe pre-eclampsia who is in a critical care setting where delivery is planned within 24 hours
   c. Woman with severe hypertension who has had a seizure previously
   d. Woman with mild-to-moderate blood pressure elevation planned for surgery at term

Q2. Regular tests for loss of patellar reflexes check for _____ toxicity.
   a. Atenolol
   b. Enalapril
   c. Magnesium
   d. Methyldopa

Q3. Which would be consistent with a seizure due to eclampsia?
   a. There is status epilepticus
   b. No proteinuria or hypertension
   c. Focal neurological signs
   d. It responds to benzodiazepines

Q4. Which of the following accounts for eclampsia?
   a. Reduced placental blood flow
   b. Reduced cerebral perfusion
   c. Increased vascular resistance
   d. Clotting dysfunction

Q5. The antihypertensive drug not used for management of eclampsia is:
   a. IV hydralazine
   b. IV labetalol
   c. Oral nifedipine
   d. IV enalapril

Ans. 1-d, 2-b, 3-d, 4-b, 5-d

DISCUSSION

Eclampsia is diagnosed clinically with the development of new-onset, generalized, tonic-clonic seizures or occurrence of coma in a woman suffering from pre-eclampsia. Though there have been significant advancements in the detection and management modalities, the most common cause of maternal morbidity and death is attributed to pre-eclampsia/eclampsia.

Eclampsia occurs preterm in approximately 50% of women and between 20 and 30 weeks of gestation in approximately 20%.

The exact reason of seizures in pre-eclamptic women is not clearly established. Two models have been proposed based on the central role of hypertension. First model proposes that hypertension causes a collapse of the autoregulatory structure of the cerebral circulation, leading to hyperperfusion, endothelial dysfunction, and brain edema. Second model proposes that hypertension activates the autoregulatory system causing vasoconstriction of cerebral vessels leading to hypoperfusion, localized ischemia, and subsequent fluid leakage.

Fetal bradycardia, for at least 3-5 minutes, is a common finding during and immediately after the seizure. Resolution of maternal seizure activity is associated with fetal tachycardia and loss of heart rate variability, sometimes along with transient decelerations. The fetal heart rate pattern generally improves with maternal and fetal therapeutic interventions. A nonreassuring pattern with frequent, recurrent decelerations for >10-15 minutes despite maternal and fetal resuscitative interventions suggests the possibility of an occult abruption.

Physical examination reveals many neurologic observations including deficits in memory, visual perception, and visual processing and cranial nerve functions, elevated deep tendon reflexes, and altered mental status.
Maintaining airway patency and preventing aspiration are the initial priorities. The immediate issues include:
- Prevention of maternal hypoxia and trauma.
- Treatment of severe hypertension.
- Prevention of recurrent seizures.
- Evaluation for prompt delivery.

The preferred medication for women with eclampsia is administration of magnesium sulfate than other anticonvulsants. Magnesium sulfate decreases the frequency of repeated seizures by one-half to two-thirds and reduces the rate of maternal death by one-third as compared to phenytoin and diazepam.

Loading doses of magnesium sulfate followed by maintenance are given. Total of 6 g loading dose over 15-20 minutes, followed by 2 g/h, as a continuous intravenous infusion.

Assessment of deep tendon reflexes, respiration, and urine output is to be done (respirations are >12/min and urine output is above 100 mL in 4 hours).

The only treatment that serves complete cure is delivery, but this does not preclude induction of labor. For women <32 to 34 weeks of gestation and with an unfavorable cervix, cesarean delivery is a suitable option.

Seizures caused by eclampsia most often resolve after delivery, generally within a few hours to few days. If occurrence happens before delivery, magnesium sulfate administration is prolonged for 24 to 48 hours postpartum.

The risk of recurrent eclampsia in a future pregnancy is 2%.

CASE 5: Hypertension in Postpartum Period

A 26-year-old female, who had an uneventful pregnancy and peripartum period, presented with severe headache on 3rd postpartum day. On examination, her BP was found to be 170/100 mm Hg. There was no history of hypertension during pregnancy. No focal neurological deficit was present.

Q1. Incidence of new onset postpartum hypertension:
 a. <3%
 b. 3–10%
 c. 10–25%
 d. >25%

Q2. Which angiotensin-converting enzyme (ACE) inhibitor can be used in postpartum period?
 a. Captopril
 b. Lisinopril
 c. Enalapril
 d. Ramipril

Q3. Which of the following is a life-threatening complication of postpartum hypertension?
 a. Intracranial hemorrhage
 b. Eclampsia
 c. Reversible cerebral vasoconstriction syndrome
 d. All of the above

Q4. Which of the following statement is false about reversible cerebral vasoconstriction syndrome?
 a. Associated with multifocal arterial constriction
 b. Usually occurs 1 to 2 days postpartum
 c. Associated with thunderclap headaches
 d. All are true

Q5. Risk factors for sustained hypertension include all except:
 a. Low BMI
 b. Preterm pre-eclampsia
 c. History of chronic hypertension
 d. Obesity

Ans. 1-a, 2-c, 3-d, 4-b, 5-a

DISCUSSION

Pregnant women may experience generalized systemic vasodilation. Though cardiac output rises by 40–50%, there is a reduction in the level of mean arterial pressure by about 10 mm Hg and the least value is attained by mid-pregnancy.

During the last trimester, blood pressure gradually increases to pre-pregnancy values. Normally, there is a decrease in blood pressure immediately after delivery. The value shows a tendency to increase and attain the highest by 3–6 days postpartum. This is seen in both, women with hypertension during pregnancy and normotensive women.

Transient hypertension can occur in women postpartum after uncomplicated pregnancy cases. The reason may be attributed to pain during delivery, drug intake, excess fluid administration, movement of salt and water, accumulated during pregnancy, into the intravascular compartment, or restoration of nonpregnant vascular tone. It is essential to understand normal postpartum variations in BP so as to refrain from any unnecessary medication.

Women with previous chronic hypertension, long duration of antihypertensive treatment in pregnancy, higher maximum systolic and diastolic blood pressures, higher body mass index, or occurrence of preterm pre-eclampsia, are more likely to have sustained hypertension. About one in five women with hypertension in pregnancy will have persistently raised blood pressure (chronic hypertension) and will need antihypertensive drugs at 2 years.

The incidence of new onset postpartum hypertension is estimated to occur in 0.3–2.8% of women. The NICE guidelines on routine postpartum care recommend checking blood pressure within 6 hours of delivery in all normotensive women without complications of pregnancy. The guidelines also recommend to check blood pressure on day 5 postpartum to recognize a patient with delayed features of pre-eclampsia. Estimating proteinuria soon after delivery is usually avoided due to the presence of lochia.

Symptoms of increased blood pressure are as follows:
- Severe headache that increases in frequency and not subsides with usual analgesics.
- Visual disturbances including blurring, presence of flashing lights, double vision, or floating spots in vision.
- Nausea, vomiting, and malaise.
- Breathlessness due to pulmonary edema.
- Abrupt swelling of face and upper and lower limbs.
- Seizures up to 4 weeks postpartum.

The crucial and utmost essential concern is to identify women suffering from severe hypertension or postpartum pre-eclampsia, who are at increased risk of life-threatening complications including intracranial hemorrhage, eclampsia, or reversible cerebral vasoconstriction syndrome. The latter, a cerebrovascular disorder, shows multifocal arterial constriction and dilation, which frequently develops 3–14 postpartum. The syndrome is usually accompanied with thunderclap headaches.

Management of postpartum hypertension is extremely important (**Flowchart 1**). Research on the use of antihypertensive medications for postpartum use is very limited. High protein-binding agents and those with less lipid solubility are less likely to be transferred in breast milk. As recommended by NICE, methyldopa is substituted with an alternative agent due to its associated effects such as sedation, postural hypertension, and depression. Although angiotensin-converting enzyme inhibitors and angiotensin receptor blockers are contraindicated in pregnancy, enalapril may be safely used in lactating women (**Table 1**).

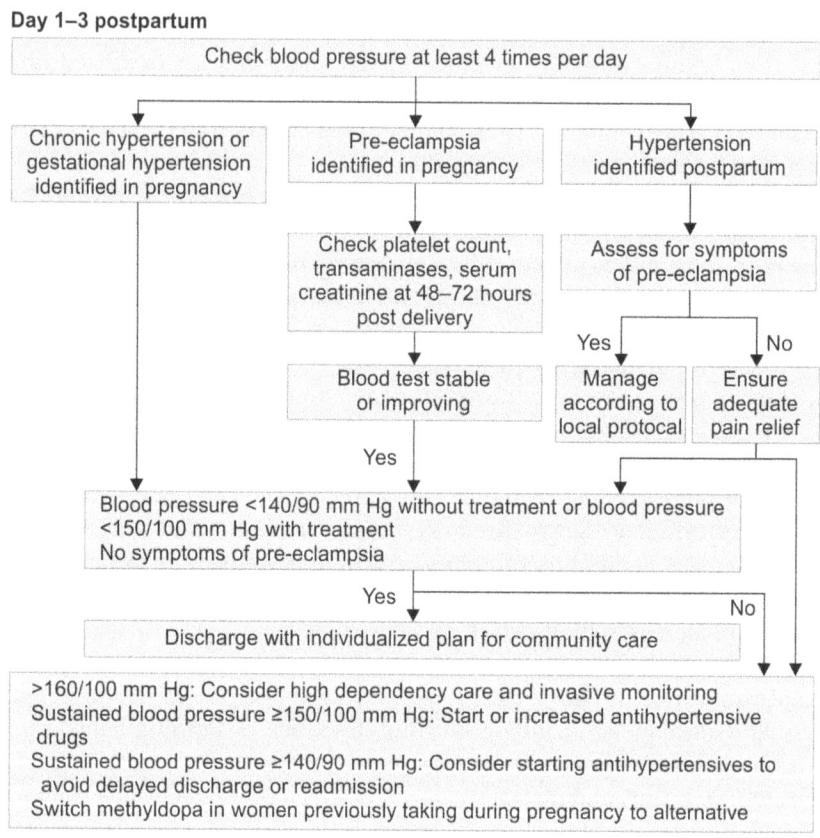

Flowchart 1: Management of postpartum hypertension.

TABLE 1: Drugs and dosages for breastfeeding mothers.

Drug	Dose	Comments
α/β blockers:		
Labetalol	100–600 mg 2–3 times daily	Only small quantities detected in breast milk
Atenolol	25–100 mg once daily	Second line use for women who require once daily formulation

Continued

Continued

Drug	Dose	Comments
Calcium channel antagonists:		
Nifedipine SR	10–20 mg twice daily	Amount in breast milk too small to be harmful; manufacturer suggests avoid but widely used without reports of neonatal side effects
Amlodipine	5–10 mg once daily	Second line use for women who require once daily formulation; amount in breast milk too small to be harmful; manufacturer suggests these drugs should be avoided but used in clinical practice without report of harm
Nifedipine MR	30–60 mg once daily	
Angiotensin-converting enzyme (ACE) inhibitors:		
Enalapril	5–20 mg twice daily	Can be used in women who were previously taking an ACE inhibitor when other first choice agents cannot be used or cardiac/renal protection is needed; excreted into breast milk in low concentrations but amount probably too small to be harmful
Contraindicated		
Other ACE inhibitors and angiotensin receptor blockers	Not recommended	Minimal data on use during lactation; manufacturers suggest that it should be avoided
Diuretics	Not recommended	Produce excessive thirst in breastfeeding women; large doses may suppress lactation

Predictors of subsequent development of hypertension in women with resolution of postpartum hypertension include obesity, high-normal blood pressure, family history of hypertension, recurrence of a hypertensive disorder in a subsequent pregnancy, and markers of the metabolic syndrome including dyslipidemia and hyperinsulinemia.

SECTION 6
Hypertension and Renal Disorders

Narinder Pal Singh

CASE 1: Hypertension in Patient with Glomerular Filtration Rate <15

A 34-year-old man came in emergency department with dyspnea, vomiting, and diffuse myalgia for 1 week. No recent infection was reported. One month before, a severe hypertension was detected by his general practitioner but the patient refused to take any prescribed medication. He just reported the regular intake of nonsteroidal anti-inflammatory drugs (NSAIDs) for recurrent headache. Upon admission, hypertension was present (145/90 mm Hg). Physical examination disclosed slight ankle edema. Blood tests showed renal failure (urea: 200 mg/dL, creatinine: 4.6 mg/dL, and eGFR: 14.9 mL/min/1.72 m²). Urine test was positive for red blood cells (++) and proteins (++). The patient undergoes a renal biopsy. Light microscopy showed increase in the cellularity as well as the mesangial matrix. Large mesangial IgA deposits were also seen in the glomerular mesangium via immunofluorescence microscopy. Diagnosis of IgA nephropathy (IgAN) with hypertension was established for the patient.

Q1. Pathogenesis of hypertension in IgAN includes except:
   a. Sodium and water retention
   b. Excessive activity of RAAS system
   c. Over-activated sympathetic nervous system
   d. Decreasing sodium sensitivity

Q2. For hypertension in IgAN, which of the statements given below is incorrect?
   a. Hypertension is primarily volume dependent in patients with IgAN
   b. Blood pressure >180/120 mm Hg with retinopathy (grade III or IV) indicates malignant hypertension (MHT)
   c. Rise in the volume of blood related to worsening mechanism of renal function
   d. Choice of drug for this patient is an angiotensin-converting enzyme inhibitor/angiotensin

Q3. Which of the medications listed below should be recommended for improving his proteinuria and control of BP?
   a. Carvedilol
   b. Frusemide
   c. Lisinopril

d. Prednisone
   e. Nifedipine

Q4. How much increase in serum creatinine from baseline is considered normal after starting ACE inhibitor/ARB?
   a. 30%
   b. 40%
   c. 50%
   d. 60%

Q5. What is the recommended BP target in patients with stage V chronic kidney disease (CKD) according to KDIGO?
   a. <120/80 mm Hg
   b. <125/80 mm Hg
   c. <130/80 mm Hg
   d. <140/90 mm Hg

Ans. 1-d, 2-c, 3-c, 4-a, 5-c

DISCUSSION

Hypertension is a frequent finding in CKD. Renal parenchymal hypertension can occur due to various factors such as acute or chronic glomerulonephritis (GN), diabetic nephropathy, polycystic kidney disease, hypertensive nephrosclerosis, and other renal microvascular disorders. Factors responsible for causing chronic GN with hypertension can be summed up as follows—(1) IgAN, (2) membranous nephropathy, (3) membranoproliferative GN, and (4) focal segmental glomerulosclerosis. In IgAN patients, 9–53% and 7–15% suffer hypertension and MHT, respectively. One of the most common causes of secondary MHT is IgAN. MHT is found to occur in patients who present with blood pressure >180/120 mm Hg and those who present with a grade III/IV (Keith-Wagener-Barker classification) hypertensive retinopathy in the fundus.

Pathogenesis of Hypertension

Following are the three important factors responsible for causing hypertension:
1. *Sodium and water retention*: Due to tubulointerstitial damage and occurrence of glomerulosclerosis, there is an increased sensitivity to sodium in the body.
2. *Excessive activity of renin-angiotensin-aldosterone system (RAAS)*: Renal ischemia induced by microvascular damage is a potent stimulus of renin secretion.
3. *Overactivity of sympathetic nervous system*: The afferent signal may arise within the kidneys. Renal ischemia is most likely a primary event which results in an increased activity of the sympathetic nervous system.

   In case of IgAN patients, hypertension is chiefly dependent on volume, and rise in the blood volume cannot be linked to worsening of the renal function such as GFR and plasma renin activity. In patients presenting with IgAN and mild proteinuria, it was noted that hypertension was directly related to—(1) glomerular sclerosis, (2) interstitial fibrosis/tubular atrophy, (3) interstitial infiltration, as well as (4) arteriosclerosis. However, it did not have any relation to the mesangial score.

In patients with IgAN, the following were found to be significantly higher— (1) urinary angiotensinogen levels, (2) higher activity in immunoreactivity of angiotensin II, and (3) overexpression of angiotensinogen in the renal tissue. The urinary angiotensinogen level is indicative of the activity of the intrarenal RAAS system. During the early stages, role of intrarenal reactive oxygen species and RAAS activation is quite crucial.

Consequent to an increase in the levels of urinary angiotensinogen as a result of increased salt retention and associated damage of the renal system, there is prevalence of salt-sensitive hypertension in patients with IgAN. Hence, it can be concluded that with the progression of renal damage, patients with chronic GN become salt sensitive. Furthermore, lowering of interstitial blood flow and hypoxia causes stimulation of the intrarenal RAAS which further aggravates condition of salt-sensitive hypertension.

Antihypertensive Therapy

In most patients in whom albumin excretion rate is ≥30 mg/24 h, a blood pressure target of ≤130 mm Hg or ≤80 mm Hg has been suggested. According to the JNC 8 guidelines, patients with CKD and proteinuria are recommended treatment with either an ARB or an ACE inhibitor. The concomitant use of an ACE inhibitor/ARB with a calcium channel blocker (long-acting dihydropyridine or nondihydropyridine) and a diuretic can also be efficient in achievement of the target BP and to decrease the amount of protein excretion in urine. As a result of either an ARB or an ACE inhibitor, it is common to have increased level of creatinine by 30%, which indicates lowering of glomerular filtration and glomerular hypertension. This physiological response is reversible and harmless. Close monitoring of serum chemistry and proteinuria in every 2–4 weeks should be recommended.

KDIGO Recommendations

"If proteinuria is >1 g/day (1B) or between 0.5 g/day and 1 g/day (2D), angiotensin-converting-enzyme inhibitors or ARBs are recommended, and 6 months of corticosteroid is recommended if proteinuria is persistent despite 3–6 months of ACE inhibitor and BP is under control (2C). Fish oil is recommended as an assistive treatment (2D)."

CASE 2: Hypertension in Patient with Glomerular Filtration Rate 30–60

A 72-year-old nonobese male presents in the emergency department with the chief complaint of hypertension since 2 years and experiencing shortness of breath. Following are the patient's vitals: BP: 168/102 mm Hg, HR: 91 bpm, and clinic BP was 146/82 mm Hg. Current medications include: HCTZ 25 mg, ramipril 10 mg, and metoprolol succinate 100 mg (all are taken once daily). The chest X-ray is consistent for pulmonary edema. Laboratory results revealed creatinine to be 1.8 mg/dL (eGFR—42 mL/min/1.73 m^2), which increased from 1.2 mg/dL.

Q1. Which one of the findings listed below indicates renovascular hypertension (RVH) in this patient?
   a. BP >160/100 mm Hg (hypertension stage II)
   b. Worsening renal function with treatment of hypertension
   c. Resistant hypertension
   d. Flash pulmonary edema or congestive heart failure
   e. All of the above

Q2. Which among the following will be the choice of initial diagnostic test?
   a. Captopril renography
   b. CT angiography
   c. Duplex Doppler ultrasonography
   d. MRA
   e. Renal angiogram

Q3. Which one of the following is a gold standard test for defining the anatomy and vasculature of the kidney?
   a. Duplex ultrasonography
   b. CT angiography
   c. MR angiography
   d. Renal angiogram

Q4. ACE inhibitors and ARBs are contraindicated in:
   a. Bilateral RAS
   b. Unilateral RAS
   c. Both
   d. None

Q5. In the patient, duplex Doppler ultrasonography reveals about 50% of stenosis in the right renal artery. The level of creatinine is normal and patient has a stable blood pressure. Current antihypertensive drugs are—(1) HCTZ 25 mg, (2) ramipril 10 mg, and (3) nebivolol 5 mg daily (metoprolol discontinued). His pulmonary edema resolved.

Which of the following healthcare outcomes can result from treating hypertension in this patient with either an ARB or an ACE inhibitor?

a. Decreased rate of mortality
b. Reduced stay in hospital for congestive heart failure
c. Deferred initiation of chronic hemodialysis
d. Reduced risk for stroke
e. All of the above

There are enumerable clues which indicate the presence of RVH:
- Hypertension onset at <30 years or >50 years of age.
- Symptoms showing worsening renal function, despite management of hypertension.
- Uncontrolled hypertension, while on three antihypertensive agents (resistant hypertension).
- Conditions such as development of flash pulmonary edema or congestive heart failure, or previous hospitalizations for any of the two conditions, are few clues which point toward for ruling out RVH. The patient meets all the above listed criteria. *Therefore the correct option is e.*

Another important factor helpful in diagnosing RVH in a hypertensive elderly patient is worsening of renal function postadministration of either an ARB or ACE inhibitor.

Ans. 1-e, 2-c, 3-d, 4-a, 5-e

DIAGNOSIS

The first four of the tests given below are noninvasive and useful in diagnosing RVH. However, the initial choice is captopril test which is used to measure the GFR and the blood flow in the kidneys, both before and after administration of captopril. Increased production of angiotensin II from renin is responsible for maintaining the GFR in the damaged stenotic kidney and the contralateral nonstenotic kidney alike. After administration of captopril, GFR decreases due to the suppression of angiotensin II, which proves renal arterial stenosis in the affected kidney. The captopril test, despite of its cost effectiveness, is not very widely used because of various limitations. In the case discussed above, captopril test is not very beneficial, as the patient is already on ACE inhibitor and has worsened renal function.

Use of high-resolution CT angiography with multislice detector devices and contrast enhances the quality of images of the kidney and its vasculature. In patient suffering with poor renal functioning, it may not be the prime choice of diagnostic study owing to the use of contrast which causes risk of developing acute kidney injury (AKI).

MRA may require gadolinium, which has an increased sensitivity for detecting stenosis in the proximal renal artery. Usefulness of MRA is restricted owing to the development of nephrogenic systemic fibrosis, thus, it cannot be used as a primary diagnostic tool for this patient.

Renal angiogram is the gold standard for studying the structure and vasculature of the kidney. However, the procedure is invasive and thus does not make a first choice of diagnostic tool in this patient.

Duplex Doppler ultrasonography is useful in providing details of functional as well as anatomical aspects of the kidneys. It is possible to measure the systolic flow velocity in the renal artery as well as the aorta with this technique and the values are compared to determine the rate of stenosis in the kidneys. Systemic flow velocity increases in the stenotic artery, and a value >200 cm/s represents stenosis >60%. Values >300 cm/s represent severe stenosis. In this patient, duplex ultrasonography is a more suitable option for detecting RVH.

TREATMENT

Most of the practitioners are not keen to recommend either an ARB or ACE inhibitor for RVH patients as they are known to cause rise in the levels of both serum creatinine as well as K^+. However, as per the studies, it is proved that inhibition of RAAS is beneficial in patients with RVH. RAAS inhibition causes decrease in the all-mortality rate, leads to shorter hospital stay in case of congestive heart failure, defers initiation of chronic hemodialysis, and lowers the risk for encountering stroke in aged population who present with RVH in comparison to patients on other antihypertensive agents. However, in patients with AKI, RAAS inhibition leads to multiple hospitalizations. Despite various odd results, RAAS inhibition has been reported to enhance outcomes in cases with cardiovascular and renal issues. Furthermore, other antihypertensive drugs, for example, calcium blockers or beta-blockers and diuretics, are helpful in achieving the target blood pressure.

CASE 3: Hypertension in Patient with Microalbuminuria

A 44-year-old woman presents for a follow-up in the nephrology OPD. She has a history of hypertension since 7 years and CKD since 3 years. Her laboratory results reveal urine albuminuria of 200 mg/24 h. Her serum creatinine was 1.8 mg/dL (eGFR: 59 mL/min/1.72 m²) and BP was 144/90 mm Hg.

Q1. Microalbuminuria is when urinary albumin excretion per 24 hours is:
   a. >300 mg
   b. 30–300 mg
   c. <30 mg
   d. None

Q2. Among the following BP goals, which one is suggested to slow her kidney progression?
   a. <140/90 mm Hg
   b. <130/80 mm Hg
   c. <150/90 mm Hg
   d. <120/80 mm Hg
   e. None of the above

Q3. As per the guidelines of KDIGO, risk of her kidney progression can be classified as:
a. Low risk
b. Moderate risk
c. High risk
d. Very high risk
e. None of the above

Q4. From the medications listed below, which one can be recommended for improving albuminuria?
a. Amlodipine
b. Chlorthalidone
c. Lisinopril
d. Prednisone
e. Atenolol

Q5. Four weeks later her laboratory reports revealed no change except for an increase in the level of serum creatinine from 1.8 to 2 mg/dL, and a decrease in the level of albuminuria from 200 to 170 mg/day. Which should be the next step of management for this patient?
a. Discontinue lisinopril and start losartan
b. Discontinue lisinopril and start chlorthalidone
c. Continue lisinopril and follow creatinine and other labs in 2–4 weeks
d. Discontinue lisinopril and start amlodipine
e. Add metoprolol to lisinopril

Ans. 1-b, 2-b, 3-c, 4-c, 5-c

DEFINITION AND CLASSIFICATION OF CHRONIC KIDNEY DISEASES

Chronic kidney disease can be defined as an abnormality in the structure and function of the kidneys, persisting for duration which is >3 months, with poor health implications. Criteria for CKD (either of the following present for >3 months) are given below:

- Markers of kidney damage (one or more):
  - Albuminuria [AER >30 mg/24 h; ACR >30 mg/g (>3 mg/mmol)]
  - Abnormalities in the urine sediment
  - Abnormalities in electrolyte levels and tubular disorders
  - Abnormalities detected by histology
  - Structural abnormalities detected by imaging
  - History of kidney transplantation
- Decreased GFR <60 mL/min/1.73 m^2

As per the recommendation provided in the KDIGO guideline: In order to analyze the prognosis of CKD in any patient, the following factors should be considered:
- Cause of CKD
- GFR category

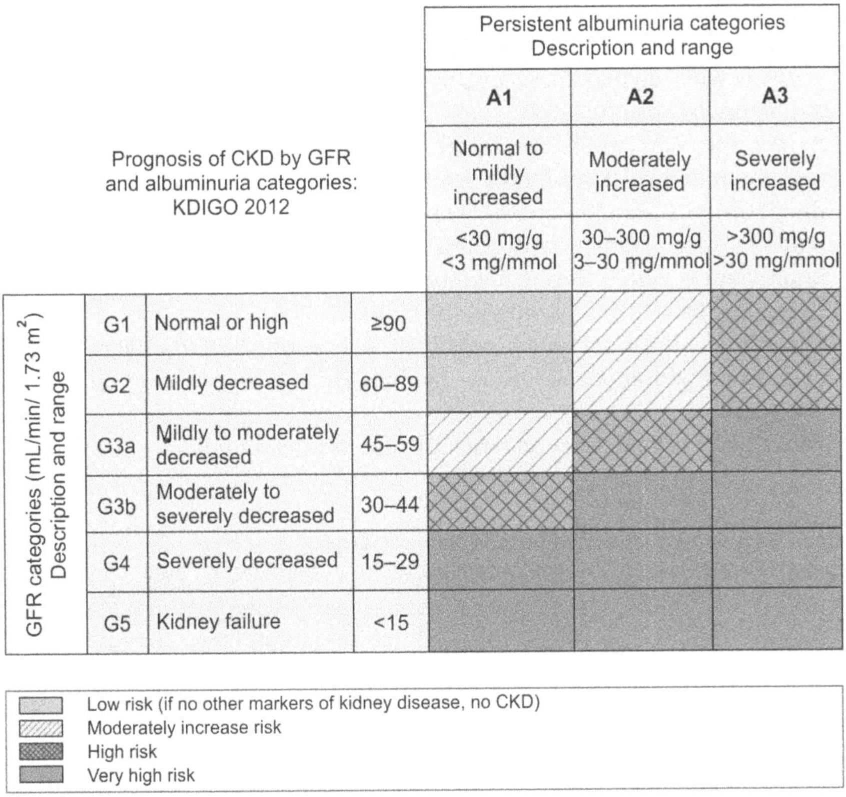

Prognosis of CKD by GFR and albuminuria categories: KDIGO 2012		Persistent albuminuria categories Description and range		
		A1	A2	A3
		Normal to mildly increased	Moderately increased	Severely increased
		<30 mg/g <3 mg/mmol	30–300 mg/g 3–30 mg/mmol	>300 mg/g >30 mg/mmol
GFR categories (mL/min/ 1.73 m²) Description and range	G1 Normal or high ≥90			
	G2 Mildly decreased 60–89			
	G3a Mildly to moderately decreased 45–59			
	G3b Moderately to severely decreased 30–44			
	G4 Severely decreased 15–29			
	G5 Kidney failure <15			

- Low risk (if no other markers of kidney disease, no CKD)
- Moderately increase risk
- High risk
- Very high risk

(CKD: chronic kidney disease; GFR: glomerular filtration rate)

Fig. 1: Prognosis of CKD by GFR and albuminuria category.

- Albuminuria category
- Other comorbid conditions

Figure 1 helps analyze the prognosis of patients with progressing kidney disease.

In **Figure 1**, it can be seen that the CKD patient is prone for progression of kidney disease. Therefore, *the correct option is C.*

Albuminuria and Proteinuria

There are three categories of urinary albumin excretion—(1) >300 mg/24 h (or "macroalbuminuria"), (2) 30–300 mg/24 h (or "microalbuminuria"), and (3) <30 mg/24 h (**Table 1**).

Blood Pressure Goal in Chronic Kidney Disease

- Sudden reduction of blood pressure is associated with chronic hypertension in CKD patients as a result of arterial remodeling.
- Hypertension can be better classified by measuring ambulatory BP and self-measured BP instead of office BP. This also allows tailoring of antihypertensive management.

- Periodic check for postural hypotension: Because of increase in vascular stiffness in the vessel wall, there is a significant increase in the systolic blood pressure while on the other hand, the diastolic blood pressure may drop down to potentially harmful levels.
- As per the older guidelines, target blood pressure of <130/80 mm Hg is recommended in CKD patients of any etiology. But, recent guidelines suggest the desired BP should be <140/90 mm Hg for patients without albuminuria (<30 mg/24 h). Patients with >30 mg/24 h albuminuria will have significant improvement with lowering of blood pressure to <130/80 mm Hg in order to slower the pace of progression in the kidneys.
- According to the older guidelines of JNC 8, lowering SBP to <120 mm Hg can be harmful and target BP of <150/80 mm Hg is recommended for the aged population.
- **Table 2** enlists guidelines on target BP and its interventions.

TABLE 1: Three categories of urinary albumin excretion.

Measure	Categories		
	Normal to mildly increased	Moderately increased	Severely increased
AER (mg/24 h)	<30	30–300	>300
PER (mg/24 h)	<150	150–500	>500
ACR			
(mg/mmol)	<3	3–30	>30
(mg/g)	<30	30–300	>300
PCR			
(mg/mmol)	<15	15–50	>50
(mg/g)	<150	150–500	>500
Protein reagent strip	Negative to trace	Trace to +	+ or greater

(ACR: albumin-creatinine ratio; AER: albumin excretion rate; PCR: protein-creatinine ratio; PER: protein excretion rate)

TABLE 2: Various guideline recommendation statements on hypertension in CKD.

KDIGO guideline			
U. alb (mg/24 h) (U. prot)	BP threshold	BP target	Intervention
CKD patients without/with diabetes (DM−/DM+)			
<30 (<150)	>140/90 mm Hg	≤140/90 mm Hg	Agent: No recommendation
≥30 (≥150)	>130/80 mm Hg	≤130/80 mm Hg	Agent: ACE inhibitor ARB

Continued

Continued

KDIGO guideline			
U. alb (mg/24 h) (U. prot)	BP threshold	BP target	Intervention
Kidney transplants patients			
Any	>130/80 mm Hg	≤130/80 mm Hg	Agent: Time after transplantation, use of calcineurin inhibitors, albuminuria, comorbidities
Children			
Any	≤50th percentile	>90th percentile	Agent: Ace inhibitor or ARB
Elderly			
• Tailor, age, comorbidities, other therapies • Gradual escalation • Close attention to adverse events: Electrolyte disorders, acute deterioration in kidney function, orthostatic hypotension, and drug-side effects			
NICE guideline			
CKD without albuminuria		<140/90 mm Hg (nondiabetic) <130/80 mm Hg (diabetic)	
CKD with albuminuria		<130/80 mm Hg	
NHFA guideline			
CKD without albuminuria		<130/80 mm Hg	
CKD with albuminuria		<125/75 mm Hg	
ESC/ESH guideline			
CKD without albuminuria		<140 mm Hg systolic BP	
CKD with albuminuria		<130 mm Hg systolic BP	

(ACE: angiotensin-converting enzyme; ARB: angiotensin receptor blocker; BP: blood pressure; CKD: chronic kidney disease; DM: diabetes mellitus)

Management of Albuminuria

The KDIGO and other significant researchers validate the use of either an ARB or an ACE inhibitor as first line of drug therapy in case of CKD patients suffering with proteinuria. Whereas, concomitant use of other antihypertensive drugs such as amlodipine, chlorthalidone, atenolol, and diuretics (furosemide, torsemide) can be helpful for managing hypertension. As in this patient, hypertension as well as

proteinuria is treatable with either an ARB or an ACE inhibitor, prednisolone will not be indicated.
- *Use of ACE inhibitors or ARBs:*
  - Patients with proteinuric CKD exhibit more prominent effects.
  - Obtain normal level of serum creatinine and potassium within 7–10 days postadministration of an ACE inhibitor or ARB along with changes in anti-RAAS therapy.
  - Increase in the level of serum creatinine by 30% above baseline in the initial 3 months of initiating anti-RAAS therapy may be acceptable and is common. It indicates decrease in glomerular hypertension and filtration. This physiological response is reversible and harmless.
  - For baseline serum creatinine of <2.0 mg/dL, serum creatinine increase of up to 1.0 mg/dL can be tolerated.
  - It is vital to consider close monitoring of the patient and careful selection of drug to avoid increase risk of hyperkalemia (if K^+ >6 mmol/L, stop ACE inhibitors/ARBs).

CASE 4: Nephritic Illness with Hypertension

A 9-year-old boy presents to the hospital with complaints of dark "cola colored" urine, shortness of breath, and headache since 2 days. There is no nausea or vomiting, no urinary frequency, urgency, dysuria or foul smell to the urine. He complains of some visual disturbances. He has poor appetite although his fluid intake is optimal.

Past history is negative for recent skin infection/rash, cough, rhinorrhea, epilepsy, fever, and arthralgia or weight loss.

Examination: Pulse: 98 beats/min, respiratory rate: 23 breaths/min, BP: 155/100 mm Hg, and oxygen saturation: 98%. Throat, oral mucosa, and nose are normal. Heart was regular without murmurs. Lungs were clear. Abdomen is diffusely tender (mild). Bowel sounds are normal. No organomegaly is noted. His extremities are warm, with strong pulses. No edema is noted in his legs, feet or hands.

On urine examination, dipstick was positive for an increased amount of blood and moderate protein. RBCs were numerous in count; 7–10 WBCs per HPF; RBC casts were present; ASO titer was elevated; serum electrolytes are normal; blood urea nitrogen (BUN): 26 and creatinine: 0.9.

Q1. Presence of hematuria, hypertension, proteinuria, and red cell casts in the urine is suggestive for:
   a. Nephrotic syndrome
   b. Hepatorenal syndrome
   c. Acute nephritis
   d. Rhabdomyolysis

Q2. In case of children, which of the below listed drugs should be considered in a background setting of renal insufficiency and proteinuria?
   a. Dihydropyridine calcium channel blockers (CCBs)
   b. Angiotensin receptor antagonists
   c. Centrally acting agents
   d. Beta-adrenergic blockers

Q3. Which of the following statements is incorrect about hypertensive encephalopathy (HTE) in children?
   a. It is an acute organic brain syndrome (OBS)
   b. Clinical presentation includes seizures, confusion, and visual impairment
   c. It causes brain edema
   d. For acute management—Angiotensin-converting enzyme inhibitors/angiotensin receptor blockers (ACE inhibitors/ARBs) are drug of choice

Q4. Which one of the following is a correct statement for management of AGN?
   a. Eat less protein, salt, and potassium
   b. Control your blood pressure
   c. Take diuretics to treat puffiness and swelling
   d. Take calcium supplements
   e. All of the above

Q5. The following are the indications for management of hypertension except:
   a. Stage 2 hypertension
   b. Secondary hypertension
   c. Hypertensive target-organ damage
   d. Nonpharmacological measures for controlling hypertension

Ans. 1-c, 2-b, 3-d, 4-e, 5-d

INTRODUCTION

The most common etiology of hypertension is renal parenchymal and renovascular diseases among children of all age groups. Acute glomerulonephritis (AGN) is the most common cause of renal parenchymal diseases. Hypertension occurs in around 60–70% of cases, mainly due to increase water and salt causing excessive fluid retention in the body. It may also lead to crisis of hypertension in some children.

CLINICAL PRESENTATION

Glomerulonephritis may greatly vary in its presentation:
- *Asymptomatic non-nephrotic proteinuria*: Proteinuria (150 mg–3 g per day)
- *Microscopic hematuria*: More than 2 RBCs per high power field in spun urine.

- *Macroscopic hematuria*: Brown or smoky color of urine.
- *Nephrotic syndrome*: Range of proteinuria is >3.5 g/day; hypoalbuminemia <3.5 g/dL; edema; hypercholesterolemia; and lipiduria.
- *Nephritic syndrome*: Sudden onset of either of oliguria, hematuria, proteinuria, azotemia, edema, and hypertension.
- *Rapidly progressive glomerulonephritis (RPGN)*: Proteinuria, hematuria, and renal failure developing over days to a week.
- *Chronic glomerulonephritis*: Proteinuria, hypertension, renal failure, and smooth contracted kidneys on ultrasonography (USG) examination.

PATHOGENESIS

Glomerulonephritis is an inflammatory process which mainly affects glomerulus, with infiltration and proliferation of acute inflammatory cells. The glomerular inflammation is initiated with an antigen-antibody reaction, either by direct antigen-antibody binding in the glomerulus, or a localized circulating complex in the kidney. The activated inflammatory mediators include flowing of coagulation factors, cytokines, and growth factors which can cause injury to the glomerulus. The glomerular inflammation impairs microcirculation, reducing GFR, and increasing BUN ratio and creatinine level. Fluid overload follows due to reduction in GFR which causes varying degrees of retention of salt and water. In severe condition, it can present as life-threatening hypertension, pulmonary edema, and HTE in some children with AGN.

INTERPRETATION AND STAGING OF HYPERTENSION IN CHILDREN AND ADOLESCENTS

	*SBP or DBP percentile**	*Frequency of BP measurement*
Normal	<90th	Recheck at next visit
Prehypertension	90th to <95th or if BP exceeds 120/80 mm Hg even if below 90th percentile up to <95th percentile†	Recheck in 6 months
Stage 1 hypertension	95th percentile to the 99th percentile plus 5 mm Hg	Recheck in 1–2 weeks or if symptomatic; if persistently elevated on two additional occasions, evaluate or refer to source of care within 1 month
Stage 2 hypertension	>99th percentile plus 5 mm Hg	Evaluate or refer to source of care within 1 week or immediately if symptomatic

(DBP: diastolic blood pressure; SBP: systolic blood pressure)
* Based on sex, age, and height; measured on at least three separate occasions.
† Blood pressure of 120/80 mm Hg or greater is prehypertension regardless of whether it is less than the 90th percentile. If 120/80 mm Hg is in the 95th percentile or greater, then the patient has hypertension.

Hypertensive Encephalopathy

In children, renal disease may present as HTE as its first sign and symptom. HTE is an acute OBS and is a result of hyperperfusion in the brain which occurs due to extreme increase in the upper limits of the brain's autoregulated vascular activity. It leads to edema in brain, petechial hemorrhages, and microinfarctions. It occurs most commonly in case of patients who maintain a normal blood pressure but experience a sudden rise in the arterial tension, also seen in children suffering acute glomerulonephritis. The clinical signs and symptoms include acute lethargy, confusion, cephalea, visual impairment (including blindness), and seizures, which is the most common manifestation in case of HTE.

Hypertension can effectively be managed in two ways:
1. *In case of acute HTE:* Vasodilator, CCBs, and α and β blockers
2. *In case of chronic HTE:* ACE inhibitors/ARBs, CCBs, vasodilator, and diuretics

In children, "hypertensive emergencies" often go along with signs and symptoms of HTE and should be managed by IV antihypertensive which causes the lowering of blood pressure by 25% or less in the initial 8 hours of administration, and provides gradual stability in BP over 26–48 hours. Severe reduction in the blood pressure may lead diminished supply of the blood to the brain, causing syncope. It may also lead to cerebral infarction or infarction in the brainstem and retina.

On the other hand, "hypertensive urgencies" in children are less complicated with lesser severity in symptoms and it can be easily managed by oral or IV antihypertensive drugs.

Management of HTE must also involve restriction on consumption of salt, weight management, moderate exercise, and smoking cessation. Antihypertensive drugs are often not deemed to be necessary post hospitalization of the child, though the child may continue to have mild hypertension for as many as 6 weeks. Reduction in the blood pressure decreases risk for cardiovascular events and decelerates damage to the kidneys. The following antihypertensive drugs can be used for the management of hypertension, such as vasodilators (e.g., hydralazine), calcium channel-blocking agents (e.g., amlodipine), or ACE inhibitors (e.g., enalapril). It is mandatory to have careful monitoring of BP for a minimum of 1 week after the discontinuation of the drug. It ensures no probability of rebound hypertension.

Indications for antihypertensive medications in hypertensive children and adolescent are listed below:
- Stage 2 hypertension
- Symptomatic hypertension
- Secondary hypertension
- Hypertensive target organ damage
- Diabetes mellitus type I and II
- Persistent hypertension despite nonpharmacologic measures.

CASE 5: Chronic Kidney Disease Patient on Dialysis with Hypertension

A 34-year-old male patient on hemodialysis was found to have high BP as compared to the initial (predialysis) BP post 2-hour ultrafiltration. Intradialytic hypertension was also noted in the last 6 HD sessions.

Q1. Intradialytic hypertension is considered as:
 a. Rise in mean arterial blood pressure of 15 mm Hg above starting mean arterial pressure (MAP)
 b. Rise in mean arterial blood pressure of 5 mm Hg above starting MAP
 c. Rise in systolic blood pressure of 5 mm Hg from pre- to post-dialysis
 d. All of the above

Q2. Which among the following statements is correct for patients undergoing dialysis?
 a. Hypertension must be favorably defined on the basis of home or 24 hour-ambulatory blood pressure monitoring (ABPM) measurements
 b. Home measurements define hypertension as BP >135/85 mm Hg
 c. 24 hour-ABPM measurements define hypertension as BP >130/80 mm Hg
 d. ABPM should cover the whole interdialytic interval
 e. All of the above

Q3. Which among the following pathophysiologic mechanisms is correct regarding intradialytic hypertension?
 a. Volume overload
 b. Activation of renin–angiotensin–aldosterone system (RAAS)
 c. Rise in the systemic vascular resistance along with high cardiac output
 d. Exclusion of antihypertensive drugs
 e. All of the above

Q4. Among the following measures, which one would you consider for management of intradialytic hypertension?
 a. Management of dry weight
 b. Restricting high dialysate Na^+ and Ca^{2+} concentration
 c. Restricting overload of fluid
 d. Avoid carvedilol for treatment of hypertension
 e. Preferring less dialyzable drug over high dialyzable drug

Q5. Intradialytic hypertension is independently associated with:
 a. Increased rate of all-cause mortality
 b. Adverse cardiovascular outcome
 c. Frequent or prolonged hospitalizations
 d. All of above

Ans. 1-a, 2-e, 3-e, 4-d, 5-d

HYPERTENSION IN DIALYSIS PATIENTS

Blood pressure measurement carried at home via 24-hour ABPM and mid-week dialysis interval is most preferable way of defining hypertension in patients on dialysis.

Home measurements: Systolic BP >135 mm Hg and/or diastolic pressure >85 mm Hg. Two daily home measurements, one in the morning and the other before the night sleep, taken the day after a midweek dialysis session, averaged over 4 weeks, are considered adequate for diagnosis of hypertension.

24-hour ABPM measurements (mid-week dialysis interval): Systolic BP >130 mm Hg and/or diastolic pressure >80 mm Hg. When ABPM is done, it is ideal to cover the whole interdialytic interval for period monitoring (44 hours with a 3 per week schedule, beginning after the midweek session).

If home measurements or the 24 hour-ABPM are not feasible, hypertension can be diagnosed as "mid-week median intradialysis systolic blood pressure >140 mm Hg and/or diastolic pressure >90 mm Hg" when the patient is believed to be at "dry weight". The mid-week median intradialytic BP is a more sensitive indicator of the prevailing burden of BP (i.e., average ABPM) as compared to the pre- and post-dialysis BP.

Treatment targets: Home BP <135/85 mm Hg or 24-hour ABPM <130/80 mm Hg or median intradialysis BP <140/90 mm Hg.

DRUG THERAPY GOALS

The arterial pressure goals should take into account an individual's age, comorbid factors, cardiac function, and neurologic status.

INTRADIALYTIC HYPERTENSION

All of the above mechanisms are linked to the development of intradialytic hypertension. Although no researches have postulated the exact definition of intradialytic hypertension, it is suggested that a 15 mm Hg rise in the mean arterial blood pressure initially is considered intradialytic hypertension. Similarly, there is no relevant research which shows the prevalence of intradialytic hypertension, but is stated as 5% and 15%.

Furthermore, adding to the above possible mechanisms, other factors like unable to reach desired dry weight, hypokalemia, high dialysate sodium and calcium composition, endothelial dysfunction, and excessive use of hematocrit and erythropoietin also have a vital role in causing increase in blood pressure during dialysis.

Intradialytic hypertension is most commonly observed in patients with high interdialytic weight gain and vigorous ultrafiltration. Furthermore, dialysis against high dialysate Na^+ concentration results in diffusion of sodium from dialysate into plasma which is a cause of hypertension.

Intradialytic hypertension is proven to be independently linked for increased all cause rate of mortality, poor cardiovascular outcomes, and recurrent hospitalizations. Currently, the treatment for intradialytic hypertension is not clear; however on the basis of general observations, the primary way to approach this is to reduce the dry weight. If decreasing the dry weight is not sustainable or tolerable, pharmacologic antihypertensive therapy is often required in most of the patients with hemodialysis. It is crucial to have an awareness of the dialyzability of commonly used pharmacologic antihypertensive drugs while evaluating patients with intradialytic hypertension. A less dialyzable drug should be considered over highly dialyzable drug in these patients, but while choosing the drug, aside from lowering of BP, other important factors such as its pleiotropic properties should also be considered for intradialytic hypertension patients. **Table 1** shows the dialyzability of antihypertensive drugs.

Improvement is noted with administration of carvedilol, up to 50 mg twice daily, post hemodialysis, intradialytic, and 24-hour ambulatory BP in hemodialysis patients. It was also helpful in reducing the frequency of episodes in intradialytic hypertensive patients. These improvements were noted to be related to administration of carvedilol in case of vasodilation and endothelial dysfunction.

In patients who are prone to intradialytic hypertension, decrease in BP with lower dialysate sodium may be beneficial as long as BP does not decrease excessively. Thus, it is recommended that regular and close monitoring of serum sodium level should be done and also for intradialytic hypotension in case if dialysate sodium is lowered.

TABLE 1: Dialyzability of antihypertensive drugs.

Drug class	Extensively removed	Partially removed
Beta blockers	Metoprolol, atenolol, nadolol	Carvedilol, pindolol, propranolol
α, β-blockers		Labetalol, prazosin, terazosin
Sympatholytic	Methyldopa	Clonidine, guanabenz
ACE inhibitor	Captopril, enalapril, lisinopril, ramipril, perindopril	Fosinopril
Angiotensin receptor blockers		None
Ca-blockers	None	Amlodipine, nifedipine, isradipine, felodipine, diltiazem, verapamil
Vasodilators		Hydralazine, minoxidil

KEY POINTS

- In comparison to pre- and post-dialysis measurement of BP, diagnosis of hypertension is better made by using home BP recordings or interdialytic ambulatory BP recordings.
- Volume overload is a crucial factor while treating hypertension. Erythropoietin-induced hypertension and untreated sleep apnea are other important factors which cause hypertension.
- Limited dietary intake of salt and individualizing dialysate sodium prescription may improve the feasibility of achieving dry weight.
- Probing dry weight can improve BP among hypertensive HD patients.
- Target "dry weight" can be achieved by undertaking clinical assessment of edema, fluid in lungs, JVP, and serous cavities, blood pressure, chest X-ray, and echocardiography. It is possible to achieve it from 3 weeks to 6 weeks in adults and from 12 to 14 weeks in aged population.
- Delivery of dialysis of at least 4 hours duration three in a week may facilitate volume and control hypertension.
- Hypertension is often controlled by antihypertensive drugs which aid in volume control. Diuretics do not have a major role in patients with end-stage renal disease. Beta-blockers can be preferred as compared to other agents.

SECTION 7
Cerebrovascular Associations

Vitull Gupta

CASE 1: Hypertension in Acute Hemorrhagic Stroke

A 70-year-old man was brought to the emergency department (ED) in unconscious state. Relatives gave history of sudden severe headache for which patient took paracetamol 650 mg, but headache increased and was accompanied by vomiting. After vomiting, patient felt dizzy with weakness of left side of body and there was loss of consciousness and patient collapsed. Relatives rushed the patient to ED. There is a history of hypertension for which patient took irregular treatment for last 15 years. Patient is nonsmoker and takes alcohol occasionally. On presentation in ED, his temperature was 97.4°F, blood pressure (BP) was 216/120 mm Hg, heart rate was 110 beats/min, respiratory rate was 28 breaths/min, and oxygen saturation was 95% on room air with Glasgow Coma Scale (GCS) of 6 (E-1, V-1 and M-4). On physical examination, the patient was unconscious and pupils were equal and reactive bilaterally. Patient was immediately transported for computed tomography (CT). CT head revealed an acute right 3.7 cm × 3.3 cm hemorrhage with surrounding mild edema in the area of putamen and adjacent internal capsule with no midline shift.

A diagnosis of hypertension with acute hemorrhagic stroke was made.
Calculated intracerebral hemorrhage (ICH) score was 1 point at admission.
[GCS score (5–12): 1 point, ICH volume (<30 cm^3): 0 point, intraventricular hemorrhage (IVH) (No): 0 point, supratentorial origin of ICH (No): 0 point, age (younger than 80 years): 0 point]

Laboratory investigations: Complete blood count, coagulation parameters [fibrinogen, PT, PTT, international normalized ratio (INR)], serum electrolytes, renal function tests, liver function tests, ECG, Echo, and chest X-ray were ordered.

Patient was shifted to ICU for management.

Q1. What is the most common cause of acute hemorrhagic stroke?
  a. Hypertension
  b. Trauma
  c. Drugs
  d. AV malformations

Q2. What is the most important diagnostic modality in acute hemorrhagic stroke?
  a. MRI head
  b. Lumbar puncture
  c. CT scan head
  d. EEG

Q3. What should be the target blood pressure achieved?
   a. >180 mm Hg systolic
   b. >160 mm Hg systolic
   c. About 130 mm Hg mean blood pressure
   d. All of the above

Q4. Evidence-based medical therapy for ICH is:
   a. Blood pressure reduction
   b. Intracranial pressure management
   c. Seizure management
   d. All of the above

Q5. Most important factor for prognosis in patients with hemorrhagic stroke is:
   a. Clinical features
   b. Temperature
   c. Blood glucose
   d. Intracerebral hemorrhage score

Ans. 1-a, 2-c, 3-c, 4-d, 5-d

INTRODUCTION

Stroke is a clinical syndrome of presumed vascular origin characterized by rapidly developing signs of focal or global disturbance of cerebral functions which last for >24 hours or lead to death.

It may be ischemic or hemorrhagic in nature. The patients may present with a wide variety of features clinically owing to the complicated structure and vasculature of the brain. Spontaneous thrombosis of cerebral vessels or thrombosis due to an embolus in proximal arteries or the heart results in an ischemic stroke. Direct bleeding into or around the brain results in ICH. Neurologic manifestations are caused due to mass effect on neural structures, elevated intracranial pressure (ICP), or from the toxic effects of blood itself.

EPIDEMIOLOGY

Epidemiological studies reveal that only 8–18% of strokes are hemorrhagic in nature and these are less common than ischemic stroke. The mortality rates are very high in hemorrhagic stroke, with spontaneous, nontraumatic ICH remaining the most significant cause of morbidity and mortality. Only 38% of the hemorrhagic stroke patients survive the first year. World Health Organization studies show that around 15 million people experience stroke across the globe every year and almost 5 million cases are fatal while another 5 million of them remain disabled forever.

PATHOPHYSIOLOGY

The etiology of ICH decides whether it is primary or secondary in origin, where primary causes contribute to about 85% of the cases:
- Primary: ICH is classified as primary when it originates from—
  - Spontaneous rupture of small arterioles damaged by chronic hypertension.
  - Cerebral amyloid angiopathy
- Secondary: Secondary ICH is associated with—
  - Vascular malformations
  - Bleeding related to an ischemic stroke
  - Tumors
  - Abnormal coagulation
  - Trauma
  - Vasculitis

In approximately 40% of the cases, blood may also extend into the ventricles IVH. The prognosis is considerably worse as IVH potentially leads to neurological death related to acute obstructive hydrocephalus.

Most common sites are the basal ganglia (especially the putamen), thalamus, cerebellum, and pons as the small arteries in these areas seem most prone to hypertension-induced vascular injury. Usually causes of hemorrhage in nonhypertensive patients include hemorrhagic disorders, neoplasms, iatrogenic anticoagulation, cerebral amyloidosis, cocaine abuse, and vascular malformations. Hemorrhage extends between the planes of white-matter cleavage associated with very less destruction and leads to brain injury by pressure produced by the mass effect of the hematoma and increase in ICP.

Hypertensive intraparenchymal hemorrhages develop over a period of 30-90 minutes duration and those associated with anticoagulant therapy may evolve for as long as 24-48 hours duration.

CLINICAL MANIFESTATIONS

Generalized symptoms of ICH include acute onset of neurological deficit typically worsening steadily over 30-90 minutes, nausea, vomiting, headache, seizures, altered level of consciousness/mental status. Deep coma is more common with hemorrhagic stroke than with ischemic stroke. Symptoms alone are not specific but patients with hemorrhagic stroke are more ill than those with ischemic stroke. Most often, ICH occurs when the patient is awake and sometimes when stressed or on exertion.

Seizures occur in up to 28% of hemorrhagic strokes, generally at the onset of the ICH or within the first 24 hours. Hypertension, particularly systolic blood pressure >220 mm Hg, is commonly a prominent finding in hemorrhagic stroke. The increased systolic blood pressure is associated with increased likelihood of hematoma expansion, neurological deterioration and death, and dependency after ICH.

The type of deficit depends upon the area of brain involved:
- *Putamen*: Contralateral hemiparesis, contralateral sensory loss, contralateral conjugate gaze paresis, homonymous hemianopia, aphasia, neglect, or apraxia.
  - *Thalamus*: Contralateral sensory loss, contralateral hemiparesis, gaze paresis, homonymous hemianopia, miosis, aphasia, or confusion.
  - *Lobar*: Contralateral hemiparesis or sensory loss, contralateral conjugate gaze paresis, homonymous hemianopia, abulia, aphasia, neglect, or apraxia.
  - *Caudate nucleus*: Contralateral hemiparesis, contralateral conjugate gaze paresis, or confusion.
  - *Brainstem*: Quadriparesis, facial weakness, lower level of consciousness, gaze paresis, ocular bobbing, miosis, or autonomic instability.
  - *Cerebellum*: Ipsilateral ataxia, facial weakness, sensory loss; gaze paresis, skew deviation, miosis, or lower level of consciousness.

Intracerebral hemorrhage may present as many other stroke syndromes ranging from mild headache to neurologic devastation or may present as a new-onset seizure.

DIAGNOSIS

Clinical Presentation

From clinical presentation, it is sometimes impossible to know if it is ischemia or hemorrhage. Symptoms suggestive of ICH include emesis, increased systolic BP (>220 mm Hg), acute headache, coma or lower consciousness level, and symptom progression over minutes or hours. None of these findings are specific and thus, neuroimaging becomes mandatory.

Neuroimaging

Basic neuroimaging with magnetic resonance imaging (MRI) or CT is recommended to differentiate between ischemic stroke and ICH. For the patients who cannot tolerate MRI or have contraindications for MRI such as those with pacemakers, aneurysm clips or other ferromagnetic materials in their bodies are recommended a CT examination. CT is more easily accessible for patients who require special equipment for life support.

Advanced neuroimaging techniques such as CT angiography (CTA) and contrast-enhanced CT assist in diagnosing patients who are at risk for hematoma expansion. Techniques like CTA, CT venography, contrast-enhanced CT, contrast enhanced MRI, magnetic resonance angiography, magnetic resonance venography, and catheter angiography can be used to evaluate underlying structural lesions such as vascular malformations and tumors in cases of clinical or radiological suspicion.

Laboratory tests should include a metabolic panel, a complete blood count, and coagulation studies in those who are on anticoagulants therapy prothrombin time or INR and an activated partial thromboplastin time.

MANAGEMENT

Intracerebral hemorrhage is a medical emergency and early diagnosis and management is crucial, because early neurological deterioration is common in the first few hours with high rate of poor long-term prognosis. Despite ongoing attempts to find effective interventions based on pathophysiological understanding of this disease, options are limited and outcomes remain poor. Evidence-based medical therapies for ICH are limited to guidelines or options regarding basic life support, blood pressure reduction, ICP monitoring, osmotherapy with adequate fluid resuscitation, fever and glycemic control, seizure management and care in a specialized stroke or neurological intensive care unit.

A baseline severity score should be performed for risk stratification which helps in devising the management strategies.

Patients with ICH are frequently medically and neurologically unstable, particularly within the first few days after onset. The standard of care should include regular vital signs check-up and constant cardiopulmonary evaluations along with neurological assessments. Continuous intra-arterial BP monitoring should be considered in patients on IV vasoactive medications. Patients who are having lower consciousness levels and poor airway protection may need endotracheal intubation. Patients with ICH are highly susceptible to thromboembolic disease. Intermittent pneumatic compression along with elastic stockings decreased the occurrence of asymptomatic deep vein thrombosis (DVT) post ICH in contrast to elastic stockings alone (4.7% vs. 15.9%) without pneumatic compression.

Blood Pressure Control

Ideal value for BP has not been given for acute hemorrhagic stroke patients by any controlled study. Indications show that very high levels of blood pressure lead to rebleeding and expansion hematoma. Intensive BP lowering (target BP <140 mm Hg systolic) early in the treatment of patients with ICH appears to decrease the absolute growth of hematomas.

Intravenous beta blockers (e.g., labetalol) and angiotensin-converting enzyme inhibitors (ACE inhibitors) such as enalapril, nicardipine, and hydralazine are administered in acute setting. Since nitroprusside may raise ICP, it is avoided. The speed and degree of BP reduction will vary according to the agent, its mode of delivery (bolus versus infusion), and clinical features. So, the therapeutic agent to be recommended should consider many factors including practicability, pharmacological profile, adverse effects, and cost.

For ICH patients who present with systolic blood pressure >220 mm Hg, it may be reasonable to consider aggressive reduction of BP with a continuous intravenous infusion and frequent monitoring of BP. In patients with systolic values from 150 mm Hg to 220 mm Hg and without contraindication to acute BP treatment, aggressive decrease of systolic blood pressure to 140 mm Hg is considered safe and may also prove efficient in improving functional outcome.

Management of Seizures

The frequency of clinical seizures early (within 1 week) after ICH is as high as 16%, with the majority occurring at or near onset. Cortical involvement of ICH is the most crucial risk factor for early seizures. Clinical seizures or electrographic seizures in patients with an altered mental status should be treated with antiseizure drugs. In ICH patients with depressed mental status that is disproportionate to the degree of brain injury, continuous EEG monitoring should be considered. Prophylactic antiseizure medication is not recommended since the prophylactic anticonvulsant medication has not been shown to be beneficial. The approach to treatment of post stroke seizures is similar to that of partial-onset seizures due to other cerebral lesions and these seizures usually respond well to monotherapy. The patients for whom this treatment is indicated should immediately be administered a benzodiazepine, lorazepam or diazepam, to attain rapid seizure control. Long-term control of seizure can be achieved by the additional administration of phenytoin or fosphenytoin. Because of their favorable tolerability profile, the newer generations of anticonvulsant agents hold a great promise in treating elderly patients. Up to 10% of young patients with ICH, of age between 18 years and 50 years, encounter epilepsy. The degree of severity of the stroke, location of the hematoma in the cortex, and the late onset of initial seizures are the risk factors for epilepsy. No studies have proved that early administration of antiseizure medications prevents lesion-related epilepsy.

Temperature Management

Fever may occur frequently after ICH; the duration of fever is related to outcome and seems to be an independent criterion to decide the prognosis. It may also be associated with growth of hematoma and maintenance of normothermia has not been clearly shown to be beneficial to outcome. Several guidelines have suggested that treatment of fever after ICH may be reasonable.

Glucose Management

High blood glucose in patients of ICH increases risk of mortality and poor outcome, independent of the presence of diabetes mellitus. Guidelines recommend that glucose should be monitored and both hyperglycemia and hypoglycemia should be avoided.

Intracranial Pressure Control

Increased ICP may result from the hematoma itself, from surrounding edema or from both. There are limited data available regarding the frequency of ICP and its management in ICH patients. The frequency of increased ICP in patients with ICH is not known. Raising the head of the patient's bed up to 30° improves jugular venous outflow and decreases ICP. Care should be taken so that the head is midline and not turned sideways. Provide analgesia and sedation as required. More aggressive therapies, such as osmotic therapy (i.e., mannitol, hypertonic saline), barbiturate anesthesia, and neuromuscular blockage, generally require concomitant monitoring of ICP and BP with an ICP monitor to maintain adequate cerebral perfusion pressure of >70 mm Hg.

A randomized, controlled study of mannitol in ICH did not show any difference in disability or death at 3 months. Hyperventilation [partial pressure of carbon dioxide ($PaCO_2$) of 25 to 30 mm Hg) is not recommended, because its effect is transient, it reduces cerebral blood flow, and may result in rebound elevated ICP. Glucocorticoids are not effective and result in higher rates of complications with poorer outcomes.

Hemostatic Therapy

The recent treatment of interest is the administration of hemostatic therapy with recombinant activated factor VII (rFVIIa) to stop ongoing hemorrhage or prevent hematoma expansion; however, no research till date advocates the off-label use of rFVIIa. A preliminary study of rFVIIa therapy presented with lower mortality and improved functional outcomes. Yet the results of a larger randomized trial did not reveal any overall benefit from this treatment. Hemostatic therapy with rFVIIa though decreased hematoma expansion, but could not improve survival or functional outcome.

Invasive Therapy

Surgery for the complete removal of the hematoma is a potential treatment for hemorrhagic stroke. The role of surgical treatment for the supratentorial ICH is still questionable. Supratentorial hematoma evacuation in deteriorating patients might be considered as a lifesaving measure or DC with or without hematoma evacuation might reduce mortality for patients with supratentorial ICH who are in a coma, have large hematomas with significant midline shift or have elevated ICP refractory to medical management. Immediate surgical evacuation of hematoma is ideal in patients with cerebellar hemorrhage, who are deteriorating neurologically or those with compression of brainstem and/or hydrocephalus due to ventricular obstruction. Ventricular drainage is not recommended as the first line of treatment in such patients, surgical removal is the preferred treatment approach. It is not clear if minimally invasive clot evacuation in combination with stereotactic or endoscopic aspiration with or without use of thrombolytic agents produces favorable results.

PREVENTION OF RECURRENT INTRACEREBRAL HEMORRHAGE

Risk factors for ICH recurrence are lobar location of the initial ICH, old age, presence and number of microbleeds on gradient echo MRI, ongoing anticoagulation, and presence of apolipoprotein E ε2 or ε4 alleles.

Hypertension: BP should be controlled in all ICH patients and the measures to control BP should begin immediately after ICH onset. A long-term goal of systolic BP <130 mm Hg and 80 mm Hg diastolic BP is reasonable.

Lifestyle modifications, including avoidance of alcohol use greater than two drinks per day, tobacco use and illicit drug use, as well as treatment of obstructive sleep apnea, are probably beneficial.

PROGNOSIS

Population-based studies show that majority of the patients present with small ICHs that are readily survivable with good medical care suggesting that excellent medical care likely has a potent, direct impact on ICH morbidity and mortality.

The prognosis in hemorrhagic stroke patients varies based on the intensity of stroke and the location and size of the hemorrhage. Lower Glasgow Coma Scale (GCS) scores are associated with poorer prognosis and higher mortality rates. An increased blood volume while the patient presents to the specialist also leads to a poorer prognosis. Growth of hematoma volume is associated with a poorer functional outcome and very high mortality rate.

For predicting outcome in hemorrhagic stroke, the intracerebral hemorrhage score is the most commonly used instrument. The score is calculated as shown in **Tables 1 and 2.**

A study by Hemphill et al. revealed that all patients with an Intracerebral Hemorrhage score of 0 survived, while those with a score of 5 died; the 30-day mortality increased steadily with the score.

The following are the other prognostic factors:
- Nonaneurysmal perimesencephalic stroke has a less severe clinical course and, in general, a better prognosis.
- The presence of blood in the ventricles is associated with a higher mortality rate; in one study, the presence of intraventricular blood at presentation was associated with a mortality increase of >2-fold.

TABLE 1: Intracerebral Hemorrhage (ICH) score.

GCS	3–4	2
	5–12	1
	13–15	0
ICH volume	≥30 cm^3	1
	<30 cm^3	0
Intraventricular hemorrhage	Yes	1
	No	0
Location	Infratentorial	1
	Supratentorial	0
Age	≥80 years	1
	<80 years	0

TABLE 2: Intracerebral Hemorrhage (ICH) score and 30-day mortality.

ICH score	30-day mortality
0	0%
1	13%
2	26%
3	72%
4	97%
5	100%
6	100%

- Patients with oral anticoagulation-associated ICH have higher mortality rates and poorer functional outcomes.

CONCLUSION

No effective targeted therapy for hemorrhagic stroke exists yet. ICH is a medical emergency and early diagnosis and management is crucial. The medical management of ICH patients comprises of basic life support, lowering BP, monitoring of ICP, osmotherapy with enough fluid resuscitation, and fever and glycemic control. It should also aim at prevention of seizures and adequate medical care in a specialized stroke or neurological intensive care unit. The studies of rFVIIa have not shown beneficial results as yet. Surgical removal of hematoma, either via open craniotomy or endoscopy, may be indicated in some patients that may improve long-term prognosis. The prognosis varies based on the severity, location, and size of ICH.

SUGGESTED READING

1. Hemphill JC 3rd, Greenberg SM, Anderson CS, et al. Guidelines for the management of spontaneous intracerebral hemorrhage: a guideline for healthcare professionals from the American Heart Association/American Stroke Association. Stroke. 2015;46(7):2032-60.
2. Liebeskind DS. (2019). Hemorrhagic stroke. [online] Available from https://emedicine.medscape.com/article/1916662-overview [Last accessed December, 2019].
3. World Health Organization. Cerebrovascular Diseases: A Clinical and Research Classification. Geneva: WHO; 1978.
4. Broderick J, Connolly S, Feldmann E, et al. Guidelines for the management of spontaneous intracerebral hemorrhage in adults: 2007 update: a guideline from the American Heart Association/American Stroke Association Stroke Council, High Blood Pressure Research Council, and the Quality of Care and Outcomes in Research Interdisciplinary Working Group. Circulation. 2007;116(16):e391-413.
5. Dennis MS, Burn JP, Sandercock PA, et al. Long-term survival after first-ever stroke: the Oxfordshire Community Stroke Project. Stroke. 1993;24(6):796-800.
6. MacKay J, Mensah GA. Global burden of stroke. The Atlas of Heart Disease and Stroke. Geneva: World Health Organization.
7. Rincon F, Mayer SA. Clinical review: Critical care management of spontaneous intracerebral hemorrhage. Crit Care. 2008;12(6):237.
8. Goldstein LB, Simel DL. Is this patient having a stroke? JAMA. 2005;293(19):2391-402.
9. Mayer SA, Brun NC, Begtrup K, et al. Efficacy and safety of recombinant activated factor VII for acute intracerebral hemorrhage. N Engl J Med. 2008;358(20):2127-37.
10. Diringer MN, Skolnick BE, Mayer SA, et al. Thromboembolic events with recombinant activated factor VII in spontaneous intracerebral hemorrhage: results from the Factor Seven for Acute Hemorrhagic Stroke (FAST) trial. Stroke. 2010;41(1):48-53.
11. Zahuranec DB, Gonzales NR, Brown DL, et al. Presentation of intracerebral haemorrhage in a community. J Neurol Neurosurg Psychiatry. 2006;77(3):340-4.
12. Hemphill JC 3rd, Bonovich DC, Besmertis L, et al. The ICH score: a simple, reliable grading scale for intracerebral hemorrhage. Stroke. 2001;32(4):891-7.
13. De Herdt V, Dumont F, Hénon H, et al. Early seizures in intracerebral hemorrhage: incidence, associated factors, and outcome. Neurology. 2011;77(20):1794-800.
14. Kamel H, Hemphill JC 3rd. Characteristics and sequelae of intracranial hypertension after intracerebral hemorrhage. Neurocrit Care. 2012;17(2):172-6.
15. Misra UK, Kalita J, Ranjan P, et al. Mannitol in intracerebral hemorrhage: a randomized controlled study. J Neurol Sci. 2005;234(1-2):41-5.
16. Yank V, Tuohy CV, Logan AC, et al. Systematic review: Benefits and harms of in-hospital use of recombinant factor VIIa for off-label indications. Ann Intern Med. 2011;154(8):529-40.

CASE 2: Hypertension in Acute Ischemic Stroke

A 68-year-old female presents to the OPD with history of weakness of left side of the body for about 8 hours. Patient got up in the morning with a feeling of weakness of left arm and was unable to button her shirt. After some time, she felt weakness of left side of face and deviation of angle of mouth. Weakness gradually increased to whole of the arm, face, and leg over a period of 3–4 hours. Patient gave a history of hypertension for about 20 years and taking tablet amlodipine 5 mg and atenolol 50 mg with irregular check-up and treatment. Relatives took her to a registered medical practitioner who gave her some injections and tablets, but the problem increased so much that the patient was unable to move her left arm and left leg with weakness of face and deviation of angle of mouth. There was no history of sudden severe headache, nausea or vomiting or altered consciousness, seizures or episodes of loss of consciousness. Her vitals were as follows: Blood pressure—184/102 mm Hg; heart rate—96 beats/min; respiratory rate—18 breaths/min; and 98% saturation of O_2 on room air. On physical examination, the patient was conscious, well-oriented, pupils were equal and reactive bilaterally, and rest of general physical examination was within normal limits. Central nervous system (CNS) examination showed upper motor neuron 7th nerve palsy and left-sided hemiplegia with power grade 0/5 in left upper limb and grade 2/5 in left lower limb. Reflexes were execrated with plantar extensor response on left side showing upper motor neuron lesion. Patient was immediately transported for computed tomography (CT). CT head revealed an acute infarct in right middle cerebral artery (MCA) territory with surrounding mild edema.

Patient was shifted to stroke ward for management.

Q1. What is the most common cause of acute stroke?
a. Thrombosis
b. Embolism
c. Thromboembolism
d. Hemorrhage

Q2. What is the most commonly used diagnostic modality in acute ischemic stroke?
a. MRI head
b. Lumbar puncture
c. CT scan head
d. EEG
e. Carotid Doppler study

Q3. What should be the reasonable blood pressure achieved before institution of IV fibrinolysis in eligible patients who reach early?
a. >185/110 mm Hg
b. >220/120 mm Hg
c. <180/105 mm Hg
d. <130/80 mm Hg

Q4. Which antiplatelet drug is beneficial in acute ischemic stroke?
   a. Tirofiban
   b. Clopidogrel
   c. Aspirin
   d. Abciximab

Q5. Which drug is approved by FDA for fibrinolysis?
   a. Recombinant tissue-type plasminogen activator (r-tPA)
   b. Reteplase
   c. Tenecteplase
   d. Urokinase
   e. Streptokinase

Ans. 1-a, 2-c, 3-c, 4-c, 5-a

INTRODUCTION

A stroke, or cerebrovascular accident (CVA), is defined as the abrupt onset of a neurologic deficit that is attributable to a focal vascular cause. Transient ischemic attack (TIA) is defined as the clinical condition in which all neurological signs and symptoms are resolved within the initial 24 hours of insult caused to the brain, even though its radiological implication is permanently evident. When the neurological symptoms persist longer than 24 hours duration, the condition is referred as stroke.

Stroke may exhibit a variety of clinical manifestations owing to the complexity in structure and vascularity of the brain. Stroke can be caused due to an ischemia or a hemorrhage. The general cause of ischemic stroke is either a cerebral vessel thrombosis or by dislodgement of the emboli from a source such as a proximal artery or the heart. Direct bleeding into or around the brain is responsible for causing intracranial hemorrhage (ICH). Ischemic stroke accounts for approximately 87% of all cases.

EPIDEMIOLOGY

It has been estimated that hypertension causes stroke (54%), hypercholesterolemia (15%), and tobacco smoking (12%). However, conclusive data for other risk factors were not available.

CLINICAL FEATURES

Complete history and neurologic examination are important to localize the area of brain dysfunction and in ischemic stroke it generally corresponds to the artery involved.

Stroke syndromes can be divided into:
- Large-vessel stroke within the anterior circulation.
- Large-vessel stroke within the posterior circulation.
- Small-vessel disease of either vascular bed.

Large-vessel Stroke within the Anterior Circulation

The anterior circulation comprises of the internal carotid artery (ICA) and its branches. Complete or partial neurological syndromes may manifest depending on the site and extent of arterial occlusion.

Manifestations of MCA involvement include the following:
- Paralysis of the contralateral face, arm, and leg.
- Sensory impairment over the same area (pinprick, cotton touch, vibration, position, two-point discrimination, stereognosis, tactile localization, barognosis, cutaneographia).
- Motor aphasia (dominant hemisphere) and central aphasia.
- Word deafness
- Anomia
- Jargon speech
- Sensory agraphia
- Acalculia
- Alexia
- Finger agnosia
- Right-left confusion (the last four comprise the Gerstmann syndrome).
- Conduction aphasia
- Apractagnosia in nondominant hemisphere.
- Anosognosia
- Hemiasomatognosia
- Unilateral neglect
- Agnosia for the left half of external space.
- Dressing and constructional apraxia.
- Visual disturbances such as alteration of visual coordinates, being unable to localize in the half field, inability to judge distance, reading upside-down, experiencing visual illusions, lack of topographic memory caused by lesion in the nondominant area of the brain, homonymous hemianopia (most likely homonymous inferior quadrantanopia), and paralysis of contralateral conjugate gaze.

Anterior cerebral artery (ACA) involvement shows paralysis of opposite foot and leg, a lesser degree of paresis of opposite arm, cortical sensory loss over toes, foot, and leg, urinary incontinence, contralateral grasp reflex, sucking reflex, gegenhalten (paratonic rigidity), abulia (akinetic mutism), slowness, delay, intermittent interruption, lack of spontaneity, whispering, reflex distraction to sights and sounds, impairment of gait and stance (gait apraxia), dyspraxia of left limbs, and tactile aphasia in left limbs.

Clinical manifestations of ICA occlusion are influenced by the cause of ischemia, whether it is propagated thrombus, embolism, or low flow. Most often, MCA territory is affected and if circle of Willis has no defect then occlusion may not produce any manifestations. If the occlusion is at the origins of both the ACA and MCA, patient presents with abulia or stupor with hemiplegia, hemianesthesia, and aphasia or anosognosia. In some patients, recurrent transient monocular blindness (amaurosis fugax) may be the warning symptom. Common carotid artery occlusion may show all symptoms and signs of ICA occlusion.

Large-vessel Stroke within the Posterior Circulation

Posterior circulation consists of:
- Paired vertebral arteries
- Basilar artery
- Paired posterior cerebral arteries (PCA)

These three major arteries provide blood supply to cerebellum, medulla, pons, midbrain, subthalamus, thalamus, hippocampus, and medial temporal and occipital lobes by giving rise to long as well as short circumferential branches and to small and deep penetrating branches. Occlusion of each vessel produces its own distinctive syndrome like the medial medullary syndrome (occlusion of vertebral artery or of branch of vertebral or lower basilar artery), the lateral medullary syndrome (occlusion of any of five vessels may be responsible—vertebral, posterior inferior cerebellar, superior, middle, or inferior lateral medullary arteries), total unilateral medullary syndrome (occlusion of vertebral artery), combination of medial and lateral syndromes, lateral pontomedullary syndrome (occlusion of vertebral artery). A combination of the various brainstem syndromes plus those arising in the PCA distribution may occur. Cerebellar infarction with edema can lead to sudden respiratory arrest due to raised ICP in the posterior fossa.

Small Vessel Disease

The small vessel disease signifies occlusion of small penetrating artery that are 30-300 µ penetrating branches into deep gray and white matter of the cerebrum or brainstem either by atherothrombotic disease or by lipohyalinotic thickening causing small infarcts that are referred to as lacunar infarcts.

Common lacunar infarct syndromes include:
- Pure motor hemiparesis from an infarct in the posterior limb of the internal capsule or basis pontis; the face, arm, and leg are almost always involved.
- Pure sensory stroke, caused due to an infarct in the ventral thalamus.
- Ataxic hemiparesis from an infarct in the ventral pons or internal capsule.
- Dysarthria and a clumsy hand or arm due to infarction in the ventral pons or in the genu of the internal capsule.

■ MANAGEMENT

After diagnosis of stroke is made, efforts are to prevent or reverse brain injury, which include six categories of treatment modalities: (1) Medical support, (2) Intravenous thrombolysis, (3) Endovascular interventions, (4) Antithrombotic treatment, (5) Neuroprotection, and (6) Stroke centers and rehabilitation.

Medical Support

Patient's airway, breathing, circulation, hypoglycemia or hyperglycemia should be assessed, reassessed, and treated accordingly. Supplemental oxygen should be provided to maintain oxygen saturation >94%. Hyperthermia (temperature >38°C) should be treated with antipyretic medications. Extreme arterial hypotension is detrimental as it limits the perfusion of blood to various organs, including the brain which is already in ischemic condition, exacerbating the ischemic injury. It is reasonable to lower markedly elevated BP (SBP >220 mm Hg or DBP >120 mm Hg) by 15% during the first 24 hours in patients who do not receive fibrinolysis. It is recommended to bringing the BP below 185/110 mm Hg for patients being considered for fibrinolytic therapy with intravenous recombinant tissue plasminogen activator (rtPA) and after rtPA is given, BP must be maintained below 180/105 mm Hg to limit the risk of ICH. Pharmacotherapy includes labetalol 10-20 mg IV over 1-2 minutes, may be repeated one time; or nicardipine 5 mg/h IV, titrate up by 2.5 mg/h every 5-15 minutes, maximum 15 mg/h. When desired BP is reached, adjust to maintain proper BP limits; or other agents (hydralazine, enalaprilat, etc.) may be considered when appropriate. If BP is not controlled or diastolic BP >140 mm Hg, consider IV sodium nitroprusside. Hypovolemia should be corrected with intravenous normal saline. Hypoglycemia (blood glucose <60 mg/dL) should be treated and blood glucose is maintained in the range of 140-180 mg/dL.

There are numerous subcutaneous and intravenous insulin procedures which help in reducing hyperglycemia.

Intravenous Thrombolysis

Rapid administration of rtPA in suitable patients remains the first line of treatment in case of acute ischemic stroke. It helps in reducing the risk of long-term morbidity. Intravenous rtPA 0.9 mg/kg (maximum dose 90 mg) over 60 minutes, with 10% of the dose given as a bolus over 1 minute, is recommended for selected patients who fulfill the inclusion criteria of diagnosis of ischemic stroke causing measurable neurological deficit, onset of symptoms <3 hours before beginning treatment and aged ≥18 years.

Endovascular Interventions

Occlusions in large vessels (MCA, ICA and the basilar artery) generally involve a large clot volume and often fail to open with IV rtPA alone. The options for endovascular treatment of ischemic stroke include intra-arterial fibrinolysis, mechanical clot retrieval, mechanical clot aspiration with the penumbra system, and acute angioplasty and stenting. The usefulness of emergent intracranial or extracranial artery angioplasty and/or stenting in unselected patients is not well established and needs further trials.

Antithrombotic Treatment

Antiplatelet agent: Aspirin, in the initial dose of 325 mg, administered orally within 24-48 hours after the onset of stroke, is the only antiplatelet agent that has been proved to be the most effective in the acute treatment of ischemic stroke. There are numerous other antiplatelet agents proven to be efficient in case of secondary prevention of stroke. The use of "clopidogrel" has not been well established for the treatment of acute ischemic stroke and requires further research. Use of glycoprotein IIb/IIIa receptor inhibitor abciximab appeared promising in management of stroke, but a recent clinical trial was stopped due to the excessive ICH. The effectiveness of administering IV tirofiban and eptifibatide has not been firmly established, thus trials can be run on these drugs in order to know or explore their treating potential. Aspirin is not recommended as a substitute for other acute interventions for treatment of stroke, including intravenous rtPA.

Anticoagulation

Anticoagulants have not been proven to be beneficial in the primary treatment of atherothrombotic cerebral ischemia. Quite a number of trials have probed on various antiplatelet versus anticoagulant drugs administered in the initial 12-24 hours of the injury and revealed uneventful findings regarding their safety and the efficacy and thus do not support using heparin or other anticoagulants in atherothrombotic stroke patients.

Stroke and Rehabilitation Centers

Provision of patient care in stroke units along with effective rehabilitation services can result in positive neurologic outcomes and decrease the rate of mortality in these patients. Patients with suspected pneumonia or urinary tract infections should be treated with appropriate antibiotics. Subcutaneous administration of anticoagulants is recommended for treatment of immobilized patients to prevent DVT and those who cannot receive anticoagulants must be advised to use intermittent external compression devices.

Strategies to Decrease the Risk Factors Causing Recurrence of Stroke or other Cardiovascular Events

In stroke patients, it is necessary to consider cardiovascular risk factors and other comorbid factors for secondary prevention of stroke. For instance, including low-dose aspirin and dipyridamole in patients with ischemic stroke of arterial origin, oral anticoagulation in patients with cardiac embolism, statin therapy for the lowering of lipid levels, maintaining optimum level of blood pressure and glucose in patients presenting with comorbid factors such as hypertension and diabetes respectively, and smoking cessation and carotid endarterectomy in patients with substantial ipsilateral carotid stenosis.

CONCLUSION

Stroke is a global health problem and is a leading cause of adult disability. India, like other developing countries, is in the midst of a stroke epidemic. Diagnosis of stroke is very straightforward in mostly all the cases. Brain and vascular imaging remain the required component of the emergency assessment along with blood glucose levels. The goal is to begin fibrinolytic treatment with intravenous rtPA within 60 minutes of the patient's arrival in hospital. Patient's airway, breathing, circulation, hypoglycemia or hyperglycemia should be assessed, reassessed and treated accordingly.

While treatment of acute ischemic stroke with anticoagulants or neuroprotective agents remains unsuccessful, aspirin is the only antiplatelet drug which has been reported effective. It is reasonable to maintain the patient on statin therapy during the acute phase. Provision of patient care in stroke units along with effective rehabilitation services can result in positive neurologic outcomes and decrease the rate of mortality in these patients. It is also important to note that routine use of nutritional supplements, prophylactic antibiotics, and placing indwelling bladder catheters is not recommended.

SUGGESTED READING

1. Sridharan SE, Unnikrishnan JP, Sukumaran S, et al. Incidence, types, risk factors, and outcome of stroke in a developing country: The Trivandrum Stroke Registry. Stroke. 2009;40:1212-8.
2. Pandian JD, Sudhan P. Stroke epidemiology and stroke care services in India. J Stroke. 2013;15(3):128-34.
3. van der Worp B, van Gijn J. Acute ischemic stroke. N Engl J Med. 2007;357:572-9.

CASE 3: Hypertension with Subarachnoid Hemorrhage

A 40-year-old woman presented to OPD with history of increasing severity of headache for 2 days. Patient gave history of hypertension on regular medication and history of off and on headache and this headache is different from the headache experienced in the past. She had taken some medication for headache but there was no relief. Today she experienced terrible headache located in the occipital region and radiating to the forehead, associated with photophobia, nausea, and vomiting. So she came to OPD for check-up. There was no history of fever, neck rigidity, focal neurological deficit, seizures or confusion or altered consciousness. On examination, patient appeared to be in distress, blood pressure was 180/120 mm Hg, pulse was 110 beats/min, respiratory rate was 20 breaths/min, and body temperature of 97.3°F. There were no neurologic deficits. Cardiovascular, respiratory or abdominal examination did not reveal any abnormality. A computed tomography (CT) scan of the head showed a subarachnoid hemorrhage (SAH). Patient was admitted and treatment initiated and cerebral angiography was done which showed multiple aneurysms.

> A diagnosis of hypertension with subarachnoid hemorrhage and multiple aneurysms.
>
> Subarachnoid hemorrhage or SAH can be defined as an extravasation of blood into the subarachnoid space between the arachnoid and pial membrane, which renders the brain critically ill from both primary and secondary brain insults.

Q1. Approximately 80–85% of intracranial aneurysms are located in:
   a. Anterior circulation
   b. Posterior circulation
   c. Vertebral artery
   d. All of the above

Q2. The most common presenting feature of a berry aneurysm is:
   a. Subarachnoid hemorrhage
   b. Severe headache
   c. Photophobia
   d. Focal neurological deficits

Q3. Which is the most sensitive and common investigation for diagnosis of SAH?
   a. Noncontrast CT scan head
   b. Lumbar puncture
   c. CT angiography
   d. All of the above

Q4. Most common complication of SAH is:
   a. Symptomatic vasospasm
   b. Hydrocephalus
   c. Rebleeding
   d. Hyponatremia

Q5. The main goal of management of SAH is:
   a. Managing BP before and after aneurysm treatment
   b. Preventing rebleeding prior to treatment
   c. Managing cerebral vasospasm
   d. All of the above

Ans. 1-a, 2-a, 3-a, 4-a, 5-d

EPIDEMIOLOGY

Considerable variation is reported in the annual incidence of SAH from different regions of the world and a systematic review of population-based studies; the incidence of SAH ranged from 2 to 16 per 100,000. Nearly 5% of all strokes are caused by SAH. A systematic review of prospective studies estimated the prevalence to be 3.6–6.0% based on the autopsy and angiographic studies. Most of the aneurysms were small (<1 cm) with an annual risk for rupture of 0.7%. The studies also revealed that in general population the incidence of asymptomatic intracranial aneurysms (IAs) ranges from 0.5 to 5% with an annual incidence of rupture between 1.4 and 2.3% in patients with known aneurysm. The risk for rupture of an aneurysm is determined by the size and the site of IA. There is no concrete data available for Indian population. If left untreated, SAH, due to rupture of IA carries a mortality of 45% (32-67%) and 25-33% of survivors will have a substantial morbidity.

PATHOPHYSIOLOGY

Aneurysms are acquired lesions related to hemodynamic stresses at bifurcation points and bends of the arterial vessel walls. Saccular or berry aneurysms are specific to the intracranial arteries as their walls lack an external elastic lamina and contain a very thin adventitia and they lie unsupported in the subarachnoid space. As an aneurysm develops, it forms a neck with a dome. At the rupture site (most often the dome) occurs thinning of the wall, and the tear that leads to bleeding is approximately 0.5 mm long. The possibility of rupture of the aneurysm and the rate of the rupture are directly linked to the tension on its wall and its size, respectively. According to an international study of unruptured intracranial aneurysms, in patients with no history of SAH, the 5-year cumulative rate of rupture of aneurysms located in the internal carotid artery, anterior communicating artery, anterior cerebral artery, or middle cerebral artery is zero for aneurysms <7 mm; 2.6% for 7-12 mm; 14.5% for 13-24 mm; and 40% for 25 mm or more. This rate is greater for the aneurysms of equal size in the posterior circulating and in the posterior communicating artery which is 2.5% for <7 mm; 14.5% for 7-12 mm; 18.4% for 13-24 mm; and 50% for >25 mm. Formation of cerebral aneurysm can cause injury to the brain even in the absence of rupture, due to its mass effect causing injury to surrounding tissues and/or by compromising the distal flow of blood supply.

When an aneurysm ruptures, blood extravasates into the subarachnoid space and spreads to cerebrospinal fluid directly damaging to local tissues, increases intracranial pressure (ICP) and causes meningeal irritation. Nearly 80-85% of IAs are present in the anterior circulation and the common sites include the following:
- Junction of the internal carotid artery.
- Junction of posterior communicating artery.
- Anterior communicating-artery complex.
- Trifurcation of the middle cerebral artery (MCA).
- Junction of vertebral artery.
- Junction of posterior inferior cerebellar artery.
- Bifurcation of the basilar artery.

Multiple IAs are found in 20-30% of the patients. SAHs which are idiopathic in nature are localized to the perimesencephalic cisterns and are benign; their source is either venous or capillary. The angiography studies are nonsignificant.

Risk factors for IAs are:
- Hypertension
- Pregnancy-induced hypertension
- Cerebral atherosclerosis
- Vascular asymmetry in the circle of Willis
- Intractable headache
- Prolonged exposure to analgesic drugs
- Positive family history of stroke

Mechanisms and disease states associated with higher incidence of berry aneurysms include the following:
- *Increased blood pressure:* Fibromuscular dysplasia, polycystic kidney disease, and aortic coarctation.
- *Increased blood flow:* Cerebral arteriovenous malformation (AVM); persistent carotid-basilar anastomosis; ligated, aplastic, or hypoplastic contralateral vessel.
- *Blood vessel disorders:* Systemic lupus erythematosus (SLE), Moyamoya disease, and granulomatous angiitis.
- *Genetic disorders:* Marfan syndrome, Ehlers–Danlos syndrome, Osler-Weber-Rendu syndrome, pseudoxanthoma elasticum, and Klippel-Trénaunay-Weber syndrome.
- *Congenital conditions:* Persistent fetal circulation, hypoplastic/absent arterial circulation.
- *Metastatic tumors to cerebral arteries:* Atrial myxoma, choriocarcinoma, and undifferentiated carcinoma.
- *Infections:* Bacterial and fungal

Ruptured berry aneurysms cause about 80% of nontraumatic SAH and 10% by rupture of AVMs. Rupture of AVMs can result in both intracerebral hemorrhage and SAH. AVMs are thought to occur in approximately 4–5% of the general population, of which 10–15% are symptomatic. Congenital defects in the muscle and elastic tissue of the arterial media in the vessels of the circle of Willis are found in approximately 80% of normal vessels at autopsy leading to microaneurysmal dilation (<2 mm) in 20% of the population and larger dilation (>5 mm) and aneurysms in 5% of the population.

Frequent thunderclap headaches and reversible segmental multifocal cerebral artery narrowing are distinguishing features of reversible cerebral vasoconstriction syndrome (RCVS) and it results in SAH in >30% of the cases. Clinical as well as radiological findings can be helpful in ruling out RCVS with SAH from other causes of SAH.

CLINICAL PRESENTATION

Subarachnoid hemorrhage is the most common feature of an aneurysm. It generally presents owing to the rupture and resultant SAH, which leads to mass effect on the cranial nerves or brain parenchyma or sudden increase in the intracranial pressure. The most common presentation of SAH is a severe headache, which the patient usually describes as "worst headache of his life" with features like extremely sudden onset and quickly reaching to its maximum or the highest intensity. Symptoms such as nausea, vomiting, rigidity in the area of neck, and photophobia are associated to headache due to SAH. Often times, patients can experience a "sentinel headache" which is like a warning signal or warning headache and occurs a few weeks prior to the major bleed possibly because of the warning leak. Of all the headaches evaluated in the emergency department, SAH accounts for only 1% of all. Based on its severity, the patient can exhibit the following symptoms:

- Drowsiness or feeling of lethargy
- Confused state of mind
- Focal neurological deficits
- Hemiparesis
- Comatose state

Seizures may occur in up to 20% of patients after SAH, most commonly in first 24 hours and in SAH associated with intracerebral hemorrhage, hypertension, and middle cerebral and anterior communicating artery aneurysms. SAH can occur during physical exertion or stress. Despite the classic presentation of SAH, type of headache is sufficiently variable, so misdiagnosis or delayed diagnosis is common. Most IAs remain asymptomatic until they rupture. However, apart from the headaches, presentation of IA can be as follows:

- Bilateral temporal hemianopsia
- Hemiparesis of bilateral lower limbs (anterior communicating artery aneurysm).
- Unilateral IIIrd nerve palsy (posterior communicating artery aneurysm).
- Orbital or facial pain
- Epistaxis
- Ophthalmoplegia (intercavernous internal carotid artery) or progressive loss of vision.
- Symptoms pertaining to dysfunction of the brainstem (posterior circulation aneurysms).

PHYSICAL EXAMINATION

In SAH patients, physical examination may be normal. Nearly 50% of patients may present with mild-to-moderate BP elevation. In some patients as the ICP increases, blood pressure may become labile. Furthermore, post 4 days of bleeding, temperature elevation, secondary to chemical meningitis from subarachnoid blood products, is common. Tachycardia or increased heart rate may be present for several days after the occurrence of a hemorrhage. Physical examination can reveal the following:

- Global or focal abnormalities
- Retinal hemorrhages
- Meningismus
- Confused state of mind
- Diminished level of consciousness

- Localized neurologic signs such as:
  - IIIrd nerve palsy (posterior communicating aneurysm)
  - VIth nerve palsy (increased intracranial pressure)
  - Abulia or bilateral lower-extremity weakness (anterior communicating aneurysm).
  - Combination of hemiparesis and aphasia or visuospatial neglect (middle cerebral artery aneurysm).

Retinal hemorrhages should be differentiated from the preretinal hemorrhages of Terson's syndrome, which indicates a more abrupt rise in the ICP and increased rate of mortality. Papilledema can be revealed by funduscopy. In about 20-30% of patients, subhyaloid retinal hemorrhage (small round hemorrhage, perhaps with visible meniscus, near the optic nerve head) is evident.

DIAGNOSIS

Subarachnoid hemorrhage should always be suspected in patients with a typical presentation, including a sudden onset of severe headache which is described as the "worst ever" headache, with nausea, vomiting, neck pain, photophobia, and loss of consciousness. SAH may be misdiagnosed for migraine and tension-type headaches in the absence of the classic signs and symptoms. Headache may be the only presenting symptom in up to 40% of patients and may dull completely within minutes or hours, representing sentinel or thunderclap headaches or "warning leaks" and require emergency evaluation. Noncontrast computed tomography (NCCT) is recommended for patient with history of first or worst headache. There is high sensitivity of CT in the initial 3 days post SAH (close to 100%), after which it moderately reduces in the following few days. The rate of negative CT increases sharply and lumbar puncture is often required to show xanthochromia after a period of 5-7 days. Lumbar puncture is appropriate for ruling out SAH in patients in case of strong clinical suspicion and when NCCT head is nondiagnostic. Magnetic resonance imaging (MRI) (fluid-attenuated inversion recovery, proton density, diffusion-weighted imaging, and gradient echo sequences) can be considered for diagnosing SAH in patients with a nondiagnostic CT scan, avoiding the need for lumbar puncture. CT angiography (CTA) may be considered in the work-up of SAH. In majority of the cases, NCCT followed by CTA is used for diagnosing SAH. If an aneurysm is detected by CTA, it may help guide the decision for type of aneurysm repair. In case CTA is inconclusive, Digital subtraction angiography (DSA) is still recommended except possibly in the instance of classic perimesencephalic SAH. For detecting aneurysm in patients with SAH (except when the aneurysm was previously diagnosed by a noninvasive angiogram) and for planning treatment (to determine whether an aneurysm is amenable to coiling or to expedite microsurgery), DSA with 3-dimensional rotational angiography is indicated.

Assessment of Severity

Various grading scales are used to clinically assess and grade the severity of SAH. The Hunt and Hess and the World Federation of Neurological Surgeons (WFNS) grading systems are the two most often employed clinical scales. The third scale, Fisher scale, classifies SAH based on the appearance of CT scan and quantification of subarachnoid blood.

WFNS scale:
- *Grade I:* Glasgow Coma Score (GCS) of 15, motor deficit absent.
- *Grade II:* GCS of 13-14, motor deficit absent.
- *Grade III:* GCS of 13-14, motor deficit present.
- *Grade IV:* GCS of 7-12, motor deficit absent or present.
- *Grade V:* GCS of 3-6, motor deficit absent or present.

Fisher scale (CT scan appearance):
- *Group I:* No blood detected.
- *Group II:* Diffuse deposition of subarachnoid blood, no clots and no layers of blood >1 mm.
- *Group III:* Localized clots and/or vertical layers of blood 1 mm or greater in thickness.
- *Group IV:* Diffuse or no subarachnoid blood, but intracerebral or intraventricular clots are present.

The Hunt and Hess grading system:
- *Grade 0:* Unruptured aneurysm
- *Grade I:* Asymptomatic or mild headache and slight nuchal rigidity.
- *Grade Ia:* Fixed neurologic deficit without acute meningeal/brain reaction.
- *Grade II:* Cranial nerve palsy, moderate-to-severe headache, nuchal rigidity.
- *Grade III:* Mild focal deficit, lethargy, or confusion.
- *Grade IV:* Stupor, moderate-to-severe hemiparesis, early decerebrate rigidity.
- *Grade V:* Deep coma, decerebrate rigidity, moribund appearance.

In the Hunt and Hess grading system, lower the grade, better the prognosis. Grades I-III are usually associated with a favorable outcome; making the patients eligible for an early surgery. Grade IV and V indicate a poor prognosis; it is vital that these patients are stabilized and progressed to grade III before undertaking surgery.

The rate of survival in SAH patients is dependent on the grade of SAH during presentation. It has been reported that the survival rates for Hunt and Hess Scale are 70%, 60%, 50%, 40%, and 10% for grades I, II, III, and IV, respectively.

Though all three of the above grading systems are deemed efficient in determining the outcomes and timing of surgical management, however, uncertainty exists regarding the prognostic advantage of each scale over the other. To have a more accurate assessment of the SAH severity, patient's health status and general medical factors, site and size of the aneurysm must also be considered along with the aforementioned grading systems.

TREATMENT

All patients with SAH should be evaluated and treated on an emergency basis and after initial stabilization, patients should be transferred to critical care setting. Securing the airways, managing blood pressure both pre- and post-treating the aneurysm, preventing reoccurrence of bleeding before the initiation of the treatment, management of hydrocephalus as well as hyponatremia, and preventing risk of developing complications such as pulmonary embolism along with prevention of neurological complications are the primary goals of treatment in a SAH patient.

General Therapy

It is required to maintain adequate cerebral perfusion pressure while avoiding excessive elevation of arterial pressure before initiation of the definitive treatment for ruptured aneurysm.

Nicarpine, labetalol, or esmolol can be used for lowering the blood pressure of the patient when he is alert. However, if the patient's level of consciousness is low, it is appropriate to measure the ICP and maintain the target cerebral perfusion pressure of 60–70 mm Hg.

After securing the aneurysm, hypertension is allowed but the range has not been established. Patients may often need analgesia and reversible agents, for instance, narcotics, are recommended. It is also vital to correct hyperthermia and hyperglycemia which are the two main factors related to poor outcome. Prophylaxis of deep venous thrombosis (DVT) should be instituted early with sequential compressive devices and subcutaneous heparin should be added after the aneurysm is treated. Calcium antagonists are recommended as they lower the risk of poor outcomes from ischemic complications. Commonly prescribed drug is oral nimodipine. Long-term use of antifibrinolytic agents lowers rebleeding, however, it is known to increase the risk of cerebral ischemia and systemic thrombotic events. Early treatment of aneurysms has become the mainstay of rebleeding prevention, but antifibrinolytic therapy may be used in the short-term before aneurysm treatment.

Treatment Options for Aneurysms

Microvascular neurosurgical clipping and endovascular coiling are the two chief therapeutic options for the treatment of the ruptured aneurysm. These must be performed at the earliest in the majority of patients in order to decrease the rate of rebleeding post SAH. Total obliteration of the aneurysm is advised as and when applicable. Treatment of aneurysm is established based on characteristics, such as the patient's age and overall medical condition and the aneurysm's location, morphology, and relationship to adjacent vessels. Microsurgical clipping may receive increased consideration in patients presenting with large (>50 mL) intraparenchymal hematomas and MCA aneurysms. Aneurysms have the potential to cause a local mass effect, thus surgical therapy is considered to be more effective. Endovascular coiling may receive increased consideration in the elderly (>70 years of age), in poor-grade (World Federation of Neurological Surgeons classification IV/V) SAH, in aneurysms of vertebrobasilar circulation or aneurysms deep in the skull base, such as paraophthalmic aneurysms. Wide-neck aneurysms (in which the ratio of the neck diameter to that of the largest dome is >0.5) are less suitable for this treatment method. Also, stenting method for treatment of ruptured aneurysm is related to an increase rate of mortality and morbidity and must be recommended only if other options with lesser risks have been excluded. Preventive measures for rebleeding post SAH must consist of management of the blood pressure by a titratable agent for balancing the risk of stroke, hypertension related rebleeding, and maintaining the cerebral perfusion pressure. The magnitude of BP control to reduce the risk of rebleeding has not been established, however, lowering the systolic blood pressure to <160 mm Hg is considerable. A short course (<72 hours) of antifibrinolytic agents (tranexamic acid and aminocaproic acid) prevents rebleeding without increasing the risk for delayed cerebral ischemia (DCI) whenever a delay is anticipated in definitive treatment. However, delayed and prolonged therapy with antifibrinolytic agents is not recommended, as it may increase the risk for thrombotic events and DCI. Randomized controlled trials are yet to establish the role of antifibrinolytic agents in terms of overall patient outcome. Centers that combine both endovascular and neurosurgical expertise may present the best outcomes for patients.

MANAGEMENT OF COMPLICATIONS

The common complications of SAH are neurologic in nature, comprising of symptomatic vasospasm (46%), hydrocephalus (20%), and reoccurrence of bleeding (7%).

Cerebral vasospasm is still the primary factor responsible for morbidity and mortality following aneurysmal SAH. It is likely an inflammatory reaction in the wall of the blood vessel which develops within 4 to 12 days after SAH and leads to symptomatic ischemia and infarction in approximately 30% of patients. Angiographic vasospasm is more common (two-thirds of patients) than symptomatic vasospasm (with clinical evidence of cerebral ischemia). Management of cerebral vasospasm after SAH includes administration of oral nimodipine to all patients as it has been shown to improve neurological outcomes but not cerebral vasospasm. The efficacy of various other calcium antagonists is unknown. After symptomatic vasospasm is evident (with focal neurologic signs), patients are treated for hypervolemia and induced hypertension. Patients with no improvement with medical therapy undergo emergency cerebral angiography, transluminal angioplasty and/or selective intra-arterial vasodilator therapy especially when there is narrowing in focal vessel. Prophylactic hypervolemia or balloon angioplasty is not recommended before development of angiographic spasm. Transcranial Doppler is reasonable to monitor for the development of arterial vasospasm. Perfusion imaging with CT or MR are helpful in detecting areas of potential brain ischemia. Volume expansion helps in preventing hypotension, augmenting cardiac output as well as reducing the viscosity of blood viscosity by decreasing the level of hematocrit. This technique is referred to as "triple-H" (hypertension, hemodilution, and hypervolemic) therapy. Vasodilatation achieved by direct angioplasty is permanent, further allowing "triple-H therapy" to be tapered sooner. Pharmacologic vasodilators such as verapamil and nicardipine do not last longer than 8–24 hours, thus requiring multiple treatments until there is reabsorption of the blood from the subarachnoid space. While intra-arterial papaverine is an effective vasodilator, evidence shows that it has a potential neurotoxic nature and should be considered for refractory cases. Increase in the ICP can occur due to severe cerebral edema in patients as a result of infarction from vasospasm. This increase in ICP is enough to reduce the cerebral perfusion pressure. Treatment can be done by mannitol, hyperventilation, hemicraniectomy; moderate hypothermia can play a role in reducing the ICP.

Acute symptomatic hydrocephalus associated with SAH should be managed by diversion of cerebrospinal fluid, external ventricular drainage (EVD) or lumbar drainage, depending on the clinical scenario or it may clear spontaneously. Chronic hydrocephalus may take weeks to months post SAH to develop and present as gait difficulty, incontinence, impaired mental activity and must be managed by permanent cerebrospinal fluid diversion. Weaning EVD over >24 hours is not considered effective in order to reduce the need for ventricular shunting. Routine fenestration of the lamina terminalis is not efficient in decreasing rate of shunt-dependent hydrocephalus, thus it should not be practiced in routine.

Re-rupture of an untreated aneurysm in the first month following SAH is approximately 30%, with the peak in the first 7 days and is related to a mortality rate of 60% and unfavorable outcome. Early treatment can help in prevention of rebleeding.

Seizures associated with SAH occur in up to a third of patients in immediate post-hemorrhagic period. Anticonvulsants may be considered for patients with known risk factors for delayed seizure disorder, such as prior seizure, intracerebral hematoma, intractable hypertension, infarction or aneurysm at MCA, but routine long-term use is not recommended. Patients in comatose state should be monitored with electroencephalography, in view of the fact that the frequency of nonconvulsive seizures can be as high as 20%. Seizures are not commonly present during the onset of rupture of aneurysm. Prophylactic therapy with phenytoin is suggested since a seizure may promote rebleeding.

Hyponatremia can be intense and may quickly develop in the initial 2 weeks following SAH. SAH causes both natriuresis as well as volume depletion which leads to both hyponatremic and hypovolemic condition in the patient. Both atrial natriuretic peptide and brain natriuretic peptide play a role in producing this "cerebral salt-wasting syndrome." Usually it clears within a period of 1-2 weeks and in the setting of SAH, treatment with free-water restriction is not recommended as it may increase chances of having a stroke.

Oral salt supplement along with normal saline will alleviate hyponatremia, however, patients usually also need hypertonic saline. It must be noted that level of serum sodium should not be corrected too soon in patients with marked hyponatremia occurred over a period of several days, in order to avoid central pontine myelinolysis.

Intracranial hypertension following aneurysmal rupture occurs secondary to subarachnoid blood, parenchymal hematoma, acute hydrocephalus or loss of vascular autoregulation. Patients who are stuporous must undergo emergent ventriculostomy for determining and treating the ICP so that cerebral ischemia is prevented. Medical therapies formulated to lower ICP (e.g., mild hyperventilation, mannitol, and sedation) can be administered as needed. An increased ICP refractory to treatment can be considered a sign of poor prognosis.

Potentially preventable medical complications post SAH can cause high rate of morbidity and mortality and also prolong the hospitalization. Commonly occurring complications of SAH are:
- Pulmonary edema (either cardiogenic or neurogenic along with acute respiratory distress syndrome) in 23% of the patients.
- Cardiac arrhythmias in 35% of the patients.
- Electrolyte disturbances in 28% of patients.

Management with hypotonic fluids in excessive volumes and intravascular volume contraction is not recommended. In the acute phase of SAH, it is appropriate to control fever to achieve normothermia by using standard or advanced temperature modulating systems. General critical care of SAH patients may include cautious management of glucose levels with strict avoidance of hypoglycemia. It is considered appropriate to use packed red blood cell transfusion for treating anemia in SAH patients who have higher chance of developing cerebral ischemia. An optimal hemoglobin target is still uncertain or undetermined. It is appropriate to use fludrocortisone acetate and hypertonic saline solution for correction as well as prevention of hyponatremia. The relatively frequent complications after SAH are heparin-induced thrombocytopenia and DVT. Glucocorticoids can be helpful in reducing head and neck aches which occur due to irritative effect of subarachnoid blood. No good evidence to support that glucocorticoids reduce cerebral edema, or are neuroprotective or reduce vascular injury, has yet been established, and therefore they are not recommended for routine use.

All patients should have pneumatic compression stockings applied to prevent pulmonary embolism. Unfractionated heparin administered subcutaneously for DVT prophylaxis can be initiated immediately following endovascular treatment and within days following craniotomy and surgical clipping. It is a useful adjunct to pneumatic compression stockings. Management of pulmonary embolus is based on whether the aneurysm has been treated and if the patient has undergone craniotomy. In patients with untreated or ruptured aneurysms, use of systemic anticoagulation with heparin has been contraindicated.

It remains a relative contraindication post craniotomy for a period of several days or weeks and can delay thrombosis of coiled aneurysm. Inferior vena cava filters are preferably used in order to prevent further pulmonary emboli post craniotomy, whereas heparin-induced systemic anticoagulation therapy is recommended after a successful endovascular treatment.

Long-term Care

Most of the SAH survivors may have chronically disabling problems. More than half the survivors present with complaints of memory, mood or neuropsychological function, which impact their social lives, even if there is no physical or visible disability. About half to two-thirds of SAH survivors return to work post 1 year of the injury. Quick physical as well as neuropsychological examination and management must be initiated.

Prognosis

Subarachnoid hemorrhage remains a devastating neurological problem despite of the decrease in its rate of mortality since past three decades. It is estimated that about 10–15% of patients die before reaching the hospital and approximately 25% are declared dead within 24 hours, with or without medical attention. The average mortality rate in the hospitalized patients is 40% in the first month. About half of patients with SAH die in the first 6 months. Reoccurrence of bleeding is a main complication with a mortality rate of 51–80%. Age-adjusted mortality rates are 62% higher in females than in males. Both morbidity and mortality increase with age and are related to the patient's overall health status. Greater than one-third of the survivors exhibit significant neurological deficits. Patients with even good outcomes may exhibit cognitive dysfunction. Factors affecting the prognosis of SAH patients include the following:
- Severity of hemorrhage
- Extent of cerebral vasospasm
- Reoccurrence of bleeding
- Comorbid conditions
- Length of hospitalization
- Age
- Hunt and Hess grade
- History of tobacco use or smoking
- Site of the aneurysm

SUGGESTED READING

1. D'Souza S. Aneurysmal subarachnoid hemorrhage. J Neurosurg Anesthesiol. 2015;27(3):222-40.
2. Connolly ES Jr, Rabinstein AA, Carhuapoma JR, et al. Guidelines for the management of aneurysmal subarachnoid hemorrhage: a guideline for healthcare professionals from the American Heart Association/American Stroke Association. Stroke. 2012;43(6):1711-37.
3. Sanchetee P, Borah NC, Sanchetee S. Aneurysmal subarachnoid hemorrhage. In: Singal RK (Ed). Medicine Update. New Delhi: Jaypee Brothers Medical Publishers; 2007.
4. Suarez JI, Tarr RW, Selman WR. Aneurysmal subarachnoid hemorrhage. N Engl J Med. 2006;354(4):387-96.
5. Becske T. (2018). Subarachnoid hemorrhage. [online] Available from http://emedicine.medscape.com/article/1164341 [Last accessed January, 2020].
6. Bederson JB, Connolly ES Jr, Batjer HH, et al. American Heart Association: Guidelines for the management of aneurysmal subarachnoid hemorrhage: a statement for healthcare professionals from a special writing group of the Stroke Council, American Heart Association. Stroke. 2009;40(3):994-1025.
7. Brisman JL, Song JK, Newell DW. Cerebral aneurysms. N Engl J Med. 2006;355:928-39.
8. Molyneux AJ, Kerr RS, Yu LM, et al. International Subarachnoid Aneurysm Trial (ISAT) of neurosurgical clipping versus endovascular coiling in 2143 patients with ruptured intracranial aneurysms: A randomized trial. Lancet. 360:1267:2002.
9. Jameson JL, Fauci AS, Kasper DL, Hauser SL, Longo DL, Loscalzo J Harrison's Principles of Internal Medicine, 19th edition. US: McGraw-Hill; 2015.

CASE 4: Hypertensive Encephalopathy

A 46-year-old man presented to emergency department with history of severe headache for one day which was associated with nausea and occasional vomiting. Patients' relatives gave history of visual disturbances, confusion, generalized weakness and mild disorientation since morning, and had episode of generalized seizures with loss of consciousness just before coming to hospital. No history of focal neurological deficit after the seizure, but patient had body aches and pains with generalized weakness. In past, patient was on irregular treatment and follow-up for hypertension.

On examination, patient appeared to be sleepy, but arousable with mild disorientation and irritable. His pulse was 94 beats/min, regular, good volume, equal on sides, no radioradial or radiofemoral delay, blood pressure (BP) was 196/124 mm Hg, respiratory rate was 16 breaths/min, afebrile, and oxygen saturation was 98%. There was no evidence of focal neurologic deficit and plantar reflexes were normal. Because of patient's conscious status, muscular strength was not judged, but patient was moving all the four limbs normally. Pupils were equal with normal reaction to light and fundoscopic examination showed grade II hypertensive retinopathy changes. Other parameters of physical assessment and laboratory investigation values were within the normal limits. Left ventricular hypertrophy could be seen in the ECG recorded in an emergency setting. Brain MRI revealed many scattered areas of increased signal intensity on T2-weighted and FLAIR images in both occipital and posterior parietal lobes. The lesions were not associated with mass effect and after contrast administration, there was no evidence of abnormal enhancement.

A diagnosis of hypertensive encephalopathy (HE) was made and patient was shifted to ICCU for management.

Q1. The incidence of hypertensive encephalopathy accounts for how many percent of all patient visits to the emergency department?
   a. 1%
   b. 5–10%
   c. 10–21%
   d. 25%

Q2. Criteria to diagnose hypertension encephalopathy depend on:
   a. Severity of BP
   b. Neurological symptoms
   c. Rate of increase BP
   d. All of the above

Q3. Hypertension encephalopathy requires:
   a. Admission to medical ward
   b. BP reduction achieved very fast
   c. Use of parenteral preparations
   d. None of the above

Q4. The speed of reduction in BP during emergencies is achieved in minutes to hour:
  a. By 25%
  b. By 50%
  c. By 75%
  d. None of the above

Q5. All the drugs mentioned below are used in hypertensive encephalopathy except:
  a. Nicardipine
  b. Esmolol
  c. Labetalol
  d. Nifedipine

Ans. 1-d, 2-d, 3-c, 4-a, 5-d

INTRODUCTION

Hypertension is one of the most common chronic conditions affecting about 30% of the population >20 years old. Epidemiological studies published in 2000 have estimated a total 972 million adults live with hypertension and it is projected to increase by about 60% to a total of 1.56 billion by 2025 affecting even the developing nations like India. In all the hypertensive patients who visit an emergency department, almost one quarter of these experience HE while only minimal 1% of patients go into established hypertensive crisis.

Chronic hypertension is well known for being associated with high risk of cardiovascular, cerebrovascular, and renal disease. Acute rise in BP can also result in acute end-organ damage with significant morbidity. The morbidity and mortality associated with HE are related to the degree of target-organ damage and without treatment, the 6-month mortality for hypertensive emergencies is 50% and the 1-year mortality reaches 90%. The lack of data in context to the hypertensive urgency and emergency is reflected in the fact that 2014 guideline for the management of high BP in adults from the Eighth Joint National Committee (JNC 8) does not even mention acute hypertension or hypertensive urgency or emergency.

DEFINITIONS, CLASSIFICATION, AND OUTLINE

Hypertensive crisis can fall into two classes: Hypertensive emergency and hypertensive urgency. Hypertensive emergency is described as an acute, marked increase in the blood pressure (>180/120 mm Hg) in the presence of target organ damage. Hypertensive emergency comprises of a wide range of conditions such as posterior reversible encephalopathy syndrome (PRES), stroke, seizure, retinopathy, intracerebral hemorrhage, hypertension in addition to acute aortic dissection, hypertensive left ventricular failure accompanied by pulmonary edema, acute coronary syndrome (acute myocardial infarction, unstable angina) accompanied with pronounced hypertension, pheochromocytoma crisis, acute renal failure, microangiopathic hemolytic anemia, severe pre-eclampsia, and HELLP (hemolysis, elevated liver enzymes, low platelet count) syndrome. Hypertensive urgency is defined as sudden increase in BP without associated target organ damage.

The term "hypertensive encephalopathy" (HE) was introduced in 1928 to describe the encephalopathic findings associated with the accelerated malignant phase of hypertension when Oppenheimer and Fishberg noted malignant hypertension associated with headaches, convulsions, and neurologic deficits in a 19-year-old student. It is defined as an acute encephalopathy resulting from failure of the upper limits of cerebral autoregulation, characterized by headaches and focal neurologic signs associated with subcortical edema, usually involving the occipital, temporal, parietal, and posterior fossa structures. It is also defined as an acute organic brain syndrome or delirium in the setting of severe hypertension.

The terminologies "accelerated" and "malignant" denoted the retinal findings that were associated with hypertension. Accelerated hypertension presents with group 3 Keith-Wagener-Barker retinopathy which is characteristic of retinal hemorrhages and exudates. On the other hand, malignant hypertension presents with group 4 Keith-Wagener-Barker retinopathy which shows papilledema, indicating neurologic impairment from an increased intracranial pressure (ICP). Due to the presence of a continuum between the clinical syndromes of hypertensive urgency and emergency, the distinction between the two may not always be clear and precise in practice.

PATHOPHYSIOLOGY

The factors leading to the development of hypertensive urgency or emergency are not well understood. The cerebral vasculature has an intrinsic capacity of autoregulation in order to maintain a stable cerebral perfusion with changes in BP. High values of BP above the range of 60–125 mm Hg cause cerebral arteriolar vasoconstriction, thereby preserving a stable cerebral blood flow (CBF) and an intact blood–brain barrier. In chronic hypertension, the cerebral autoregulatory range is gradually shifted to higher pressures as an adaptation to the chronic elevation of systemic BP. As the systemic BP increases beyond the autoregulatory threshold of the cerebral vasculature, it results in brain hyperperfusion, due to dilatation of cerebral arterioles causing breakdown of blood–brain barrier with subsequent transudation of fluid and protein material (vasogenic edema).

The underlying mechanism of HE is vasogenic edema which is caused by the failure of cerebral autoregulation and endothelial dysfunction. Fibrinoid material deposits in the cerebral vasculature result in the narrowing of the vascular lumen. As a result, the cerebral vasculature tends to vasodilate around the narrowed lumen, thereby leading to cerebral edema and microhemorrhages. Primarily, the white matter in the parieto-occipital areas of the brain, frontoparietal junction, and the temporal lobes seem to get affected by these changes. A series of other terms have also been proposed for HE including, reversible posterior leukoencephalopathy or PRES, occipital-parietal encephalopathy and vasculature autoregulatory dysfunction. Brain MRI scans have shown a pattern of typically posterior (occipital greater than frontal) brain edema that is reversible and are most consistent with vasogenic edema. Another proposed mechanism is endothelial damage or dysfunction, which may trigger, via increased production of nitric oxide, increased capillary permeability, and loss of autoregulation leading to generalized vasodilatation, cerebral edema, and papilledema, resulting in manifestations of HE. This mechanism leads to elevated ICP which continues to aggravate systemic hypertension by stretching the receptors in the floor of the fourth ventricle. This results in a vicious cycle leading to more acute brain injury, seizure, coma, and death.

CLINICAL MANIFESTATIONS AND DIAGNOSTIC APPROACH

For all patients who present with severe hypertension, a detailed history should be taken and a thorough physical examination is important. One should ascertain the time of onset, severity, and baseline BP at home. Relevant examinations which could reveal end-organ damage and associated complications become necessary for choosing an appropriate line of treatment. Apart from these examinations, the patients' routine medications and compliance with these medications, including over-the-counter medications and recreational drugs, must be understood clearly as these may also lead to severely elevated blood pressure levels. The clinical presentation of HE ranges from indistinct neurologic symptoms like headache, confusion, stupor, visual disturbances, seizures, nausea, and vomiting. The patients complain of headaches that are usually anterior and constant in nature. The manifestations begin frequently above 24–48 hours, in association with neurologic progression above 24–48 hours. HE is a diagnosis of exclusion and other potential causes of the symptoms must be evaluated in the workup. A detailed history taking and a thorough physical evaluation is a must and cannot be replaced by routine laboratory or imaging investigations. The first key in evaluating patients presenting with increased BP should be to distinguish between hypertensive urgency and hypertensive crisis. Patients should be assessed for specific symptoms suggestive of end-organ involvement. Signs of encephalopathy include lethargy, confusion, headache, visual difficulties including blindness and either focal or generalized seizures. The examination should include fundoscopic evaluation assessing for evidence of papilledema or retinal hemorrhages. Cardiovascular evaluation should assess for S_3, elevated neck veins, peripheral edema, murmurs, abdominal pulsations, and diminished pulses and crackles on pulmonary evaluation. Neurologic examination reveals transient and migratory neurologic nonfocal deficits ranging from nystagmus to weakness and an altered mental status ranging from confusion to coma.

Investigations are focused on target organ damage and possible cause of secondary hypertension. Cranial computed tomography (CT) may demonstrate edema in the posterior brain regions and evidence of hemorrhage. MRI has greatly increased the recognition of HE, characteristically shows a posterior leukoencephalopathy, affecting predominantly the white matter of the parieto-occipital regions, better demonstrated on T2-weighted images. MRI appears more sensitive than CT and better defines the anatomy of cerebral involvement in HE. Neuroimaging abnormalities typically resolve with treatment. Electroencephalogram (EEG) shows evidence of generalized slowing and epileptiform discharges and loss of posterior dominant alpha rhythm, correlating with neuroimaging findings. These EEG findings, as with the neuroimaging findings, typically resolve with treatment. Appropriate triage of patients is a crucial part of the initial evaluation. HE can be complicated to consequently lead to neurologic deficits due to hemorrhage and stroke thereby progressing to death.

MANAGEMENT

Having arrived at the diagnosis of HE, one of the major challenges is to reduce BP without causing any further increase in end-organ failure and management should be designed according to the patient. Patients should be immediately admitted to an ICU. It is crucial to consider the baseline BP in order to avoid excessive BP reduction and prevent cerebral ischemia. It is considered safe to reduce mean arterial pressure by 25% and to decrease the diastolic blood pressure to 100–110 mm Hg. Constant assessment in the ICU along with arterial BP monitoring is essential for establishing optimal dose titration of pharmacologic agents. While prescribing medications, their corresponding side effects and likely complications as in the case of too much lowering of BP and toxic effects of antihypertensive agents must be taken into careful consideration. Worsening of the clinical condition of the patient though the treatment is in place necessitates immediate emergency investigations to rule out alternate likely causes or re-evaluation of treatment methods.

There are many types of treatment lines for controlling HE. The criteria for deciding an optimal pharmacological agent are vascular selectivity, intravenous infusion that is easy to prepare, easy titration, predictable effects, quick onset and short duration of action, very limited or nil adverse effects, especially on the central nervous system, autoregulation of cerebral vasculature, and ICP and nominal cost. Commonly used rapid and short-lived intravenous medications include labetalol, esmolol, nicardipine, clevidipine, sodium nitroprusside, and fenoldopam. Certain medicines which should be avoided are hydralazine, immediate release nifedipine and nitroglycerin.

Labetalol is a competitive and selective alpha-1 blocker and a nonselective beta-blocker that has predominantly beta effects at low doses. It produces a steady, consistent drop in BP without compromising CBF or ICP. The onset of action is 5 minutes and the half-life is 5.5 hours which makes it difficult to titrate. It is frequently used as initial therapy. Adverse effects are hypotension, bradycardia, dizziness, and scalp tingling. It should be avoided in patients with heart block, bradycardia, congestive heart failure (CHF), severe asthma or bronchospasm.

Esmolol is an ultrashort-acting agent that selectively blocks beta-1 receptors but has little or no effect on beta-2 receptor types, effective in lowering BP without significant effects on CBF or ICP, decrease cardiac output (CO), heart rate, and stroke volume (SV). Esmolol has an onset of action of 60 seconds, and its duration of action is about 10 minutes which allows easy titration.

Nicardipine is most frequently the first line of treatment for HE. It is a second-generation dihydropyridine-derivative calcium channel blocker (CCB). The advantages are its high vascular selectivity, strong cerebral and coronary vasodilation, elevated stroke volume and coronary blood flow, without side effects on ICP. The drug is proved to decrease cerebral ischemia. Nicardipine has an onset of action within 5 minutes with fewer side effects. The main drawback is its extended half-life and the requirement of considerably more volumes of solution to dilute the drug. The drug cannot be recommended for acute CHF or coronary ischemia.

Clevidipine is an ultrashort-acting vasoselective calcium antagonist, easy titratable with high clearance and small volume of distribution. Clevidipine is the only intravenous antihypertensive approved by the FDA in the last decade for short-term intravenous BP control. Its vascular selectivity (arteriolar dilation and decrease SVR with concomitant increasing SV and CO), differentiates clevidipine from other CCBs.

Nitroglycerin is a strong venodilator, an arterial dilator only at high doses, and reduces preload and CO so it may not be desirable in patients with compromised cerebral perfusion. It is highly effective in setting of coronary ischemia, acute coronary syndromes. Onset of action is immediate and duration of action is 1-5 minutes. It may cause headache, tachycardia, vomiting, and methemoglobinemia.

Sodium nitroprusside is an effective agent in lowering BP, a balanced venous and arterial dilator, decreases both afterload and preload, and has been associated with increases in ICP in addition to its toxic effects. Its dual effect can lead to "coronary steal syndrome" in some patients with coronary artery disease. Nitroprusside should be used only when other agents are not available and only in patients with normal renal and liver function. Onset of action is 0.5-1 minute and duration of action is 2-5 minutes. Difficulty to titrate to target BP is one of its major disadvantages. Adverse effects include hypotension, apprehension, cyanide toxicity, nausea, vomiting, muscle twitching, sweating convulsion, twitching, psychosis, dizziness, etc.

Hydralazine is an effective agent to lower BP, but its unpredictability and variable effects on ICP and circulation resulting in the development of ischemic areas in the brain make it less desirable than other drugs for acute treatment in HE except perhaps for pregnancy-related acute hypertension. The onset of action is 10-20 minutes with duration of action of 3-8 hours. Its adverse effects include tachycardia and flushing.

Diuretics should not be used in HE unless there is clear evidence of volume overload. This is due to pressure natriuresis that occurs and leaves these patients volume depleted. Volume depletion by itself can sometimes lower the BP.

Fenoldopam is a short-acting dopamine-1 agonist that increases both blood flow to the kidneys and sodium excretion and has been associated with reduced regional and global CBF. The onset is within 5 minutes and its effect lasts up to an hour.

Angiotensin-converting enzyme (ACE) inhibitors, enalaprilat, have been used for >20 years. Enalaprilat has an onset of action within 15 minutes and its effects last up to 24 hours, thus the onset and offset time might be too long to be used for rapid titration of BP. No adverse side effects have been reported with this agent; however, it is contraindicated in pregnancy. The adverse effects of this group of drugs include greatly variable response, dangerous drop of BP in high-renin states and occasionally angioedema, hyperkalemia or acute renal failure. The drug is mostly indicated in cases of acute cardiogenic pulmonary edema while it is contraindicated in acute myocardial infarction.

Phentolamine is an alpha-1 and alpha-2 adrenergic blocking agent that affects the alpha receptors with catecholamines. It hampers circulating epinephrine and norepinephrine action thus decreasing BP. The drug is indicated in HE patients where the etiology is pheochromocytoma. Its onset of action is 1–2 minutes and the duration of action is 3–10 minutes. Tachycardia, flushing, and headache may occur.

Clonidine and methyldopa should not be used, because they can cause central nervous system depression.

CONCLUSION

Arterial hypertension, a major health concern worldwide, is responsible for >7 million deaths per year worldwide. Hypertensive emergency is life-threatening, manifesting as increased BP with evidence of end-organ injury. Encephalopathy related to hypertension manifests as headache, lethargy, altered mental status, and seizures related to the effects of perfusion breakthrough because of autoregulatory failure. The key to treatment of HE is to lower BP. Untreated HE may progress to stupor, coma, seizures, and death within hours. Although BP should be lowered rapidly in patients with HE, there are inherent risks of overly aggressive therapy. The initial goal of therapy is to reduce mean arterial pressure by no >25% within minutes to 2 hours or to a BP in the range of 160/100–110 mm Hg. In choosing the most appropriate drug, potential effects on ICP and CBF should be kept in mind. Nicardipine, esmolol, and labetalol are excellent choices because these agents will effectively lower BP without risk of adverse effects on ICP or CBF. Other agents, such as nitroprusside and hydralazine, should be avoided because of their potential adverse effects on ICP, in the case of nitroprusside and unpredictable cerebral effects associated with hydralazine. The risk factors and factors predicting the prognosis of a hypertensive crisis are not identified clearly. Physicians should perform complete evaluations in patients who present with a hypertensive crisis to effectively reverse, intervene, and correct the underlying trigger, as well as improve long-term outcomes after the episode.

SUGGESTED READING

1. Mehrotra S, Kasliwal RR. Hypertensive crisis: An update. Indian Heart J. 2010;62:440-6.
2. Perez MI, Musini VM. Pharmacological interventions for hypertensive emergencies: a Cochrane systematic review. J Hum Hypertens. 2008;22:596-607.
3. Sharifian M. Hypertensive encephalopathy. Iran J Child Neurol. 2012;6(3):1-7.
4. Susanto I. Hypertensive encephalopathy. [online] Available from http://emedicine.medscape.com/article/166129 [Last accessed December, 2019].
5. Kraniotis P, Zampakis P, Kalogeropoulou C, et al. CT diagnosis of hypertensive brainstem encephalopathy (HBE): A diagnostic challenge in the emergency department. Radiol Case Rep. 2010;5(2):385.
6. Rosei EA, Salvetti M, Farsang C. Treatment of hypertensive urgencies and emergencies. Blood Pressure. 2006;15(4):255-6.
7. Kearney PM, Whelton M, Reynolds K, et al. Global burden of hypertension: Analysis of worldwide data. Lancet. 2005;365:217-23.
8. Varon J, Marik PE. Clinical review: The management of hypertensive crises. Crit Care. 2003;7:374-84.
9. Marhefka GD. Acute hypertension: Hypertensive urgency and hypertensive emergency. Consultant. 2016;56(3):222-32.
10. James PA, Oparil S, Carter BL, et al. 2014 evidence-based guideline for the management of high blood pressure in adults: report from the panel members appointed to the Eighth Joint National Committee (JNC 8). JAMA. 2014;311(5):507-20.
11. Chobanian AV, Bakris GL, Black HR, et al. Seventh report of the Joint National Committee on Prevention, Detection, Evaluation, and Treatment of High Blood Pressure. Hypertension. 2003;42(6):1206-52.
12. Wolf SJ, Lo B, Shih RD, et al. Clinical policy: critical issues in the evaluation and management of adult patients in the emergency department with asymptomatic elevated blood pressure. Ann Emerg Med. 2013;62(1):59-68.
13. Mancia G, Fagard R, Narkiewicz K, et al. 2013 ESH/ESC guidelines for the management of arterial hypertension: the task force for the management of arterial hypertension of the European Society of Hypertension (ESH) and of the European Society of Cardiology (ESC). J Hypertens. 2013;31(7):1281-357.
14. Feldstein C. Management of hypertensive crises. Am J Ther. 2007;14(2):135-9.
15. Bhasin A, Jain DG, Chhabra RM, et al. Hypertensive emergencies. In: Singal RK (Ed). Medicine Update. New Delhi: Jaypee Brothers Medical Publishers; 2007.
16. Castellon-Larios K, Fiorda-Diaz J, Arias-Morales CE, et al. Hypertensive emergency: An updated review. Ann Clin Exp Hypertension. 2015;3(2):1029.
17. Kuppasani K, Reddi AS. Emergency or urgency? Effective management of hypertensive crises. JAAPA. 2010;23:44-9.
18. Muiesan ML, Salvetti M, Amadoro V, et al. An update on hypertensive emergencies and urgencies. J Cardiovasc Med (Hagerstown). 2015;16:372-82.
19. Bonovich DC. Hypertension and hypertensive encephalopathy. In: The Interface of Neurology and Internal Medicine. Philadelphia: Lippincott Williams and Williams; 2008
20. Shimamoto K, Ando K, Fujita T, et al. The Japanese Society of Hypertension Guidelines for the Management of Hypertension (JSH 2014). Hypertens Res. 2014;37(4):253-392.

CASE 5: Post Stroke Patient with Hypertension

A 68-year-old female was brought to the OPD with history of weakness of left side of the body for about 8 hours. Patient got up in the morning with a feeling of weakness of left arm and was unable to button her shirt. After some time, she felt weakness of left side of face and deviation of angle of mouth. Weakness gradually increased to whole of the arm, face, and leg over a period of 3–4 hours. Patient reported a history of hypertension for about 20 years, taking tablet Amtas-AT with irregular check up and treatment. Relatives took her to a desi doctor who gave her some injections and tablets, but the problem increased that patient was unable to move her left arm and left leg with weakness of face and deviation of angle of mouth. There was no history of sudden severe headache, nausea or vomiting or altered consciousness, seizures or episode of loss of consciousness. On presentation in OPD, her temperature was 98.3°F, blood pressure (BP) was 184/102 mm Hg, heart rate was 96 beats/min, respiratory rate was 18 breaths/min, and oxygen saturation was 98% on room air. On physical examination, the patient was conscious, well oriented, pupils were equal and reactive bilaterally, and rest of general physical examination was within normal limits. Central nervous system (CNS) examination showed upper motor neuron 7th nerve palsy and left sided hemiplegia with power grade 0/5 in left upper limb and grade 2/5 in left lower limb. Reflexes were execrated with plantar extensor response on left side showing upper motor neuron lesion. Patient was immediately transported for computed tomography (CT). CT head revealed an acute infarct in right middle cerebral artery territory with surrounding mild edema.

A diagnosis of hypertension with acute ischemic stroke was made and treated in stroke ward and was discharged on 5th day. At discharge, patient had shown improvement in upper motor neuron 7th nerve palsy and left-sided hemiplegia and power was grade 3/5 in left upper limb and grade 4/5 in left lower limb.

Q1. Is blood pressure lowering beneficial in post stroke patients?
- a. Yes
- b. No
- c. Doubtful
- d. None of the above

Q2. When antihypertensive medication should be started to lower blood pressure in post stroke patient?
- a. 5–7 days after onset of symptoms
- b. 24–72 hours after onset of symptoms
- c. 2–3 weeks after onset of symptoms
- d. 1–2 months after onset of symptoms

Q3. Which of the following statements is correct?
- a. All major classes of antihypertensive agents are beneficial for stroke prevention
- b. Optimal drug regimen to achieve BP reduction is uncertain

c. The choice of specific drugs should be individualized
d. All of the above statements

Q4. What is the target BP goal to be achieved in post stroke patient in uncomplicated hypertension?
   a. <120/70 mm Hg
   b. <130/80 mm Hg
   c. <140/90 mm Hg
   d. <150/100 mm Hg

Ans. 1-a, 2-b, 3-d, 4-c

INTRODUCTION

Stroke, a global epidemic, is a leading cause of morbidity and mortality across the globe. Hypertension is the most important potentially reversible risk factor for stroke in all age groups. Hypertension is also associated with an increased susceptibility to recurrent stroke in patients with a history of an ischemic or hemorrhagic event. Unfortunately, the awareness of hypertension among people remains lesser than optimal and so does the management and maintenance. Observational studies based on epidemiology and clinical data ascertain that lower baseline BP and active lowering of BP are associated with reduced stroke risk. However, BP control in the population for secondary as well as primary prevention is suboptimal.

Important questions regarding the chronic management of hypertension after stroke are:
- Is BP lowering beneficial?
- When to start antihypertensive medication?
- Which antihypertensive agent to give and what is the target BP to be achieved?

Is Blood Pressure Lowering Beneficial in Post Stroke Patients?

There is strong evidence regarding the multiple favorable effects of BP lowering for new or recurrent stroke and other cardiovascular complications. Though how it happens is uncertain and more than one effect of antihypertensive medications may be relevant. The PROGRESS (Perindopril Protection Against Recurrent Stroke Study) suggests diligent reduction in BP can lead to reductions in total stroke, fatal or disabling stroke, nonfatal or disabling stroke, nonfatal myocardial infarction, and other vital stroke-related consequences. A meta-analysis showed that the BP-lowering treatment reduced the risk of recurrent stroke. The meta-regression analysis also revealed that, for every 10-mm Hg decrease in systolic pressure, there was a corresponding 33% (95% CI, 9–51%) decrease in susceptibility of recurrent stroke. Evidence suggest that first stroke can be averted by BP control is now substantiated for recurrent stroke also. Larger reductions in systolic blood pressure were associated with greater reduction in recurrent stroke risk. It has been suggested by recent guidelines that BP reduction is recommended for both prevention of recurrent stroke and prevention of other vascular events in patients who have had a history of ischemic stroke or transient ischemic attack and are beyond the first 24 hours.

When to Start Blood Pressure Lowering Medication?

It may be appropriate to begin with antihypertensive drug therapy as soon as 24-72 hours post the appearance of clinical symptoms in the absence of contraindications such as presumed hemodynamic mechanism of stroke. Yet, no exact information exists to decide upon ideal timing to begin the antihypertensive treatment post severe ischemic stroke. There is lack of substantial data to suggest the rapidity of BP control. In presence of paucity of specific guidelines for BP lowering in the setting of ischemic stroke, it is appropriate to follow 7th report of the Joint National Committee on Prevention, Detection, Evaluation, and Treatment of High Blood Pressure (JNC 7) guidelines for medical management of hypertension, follow-up, and monitoring BP control, with follow-up and adjustment in uncomplicated patients at approximately monthly intervals till the blood pressure reaches goal and then at 3- to 6-month intervals thereafter, reaching the target BP value within a 3- to 6-month interval is a reasonable goal. Stage 2 hypertension patients (≥160 systolic or ≥100 diastolic mm Hg) and those with other complications may need more frequent interval visits at the discretion of the treating physician.

What is the Target Blood Pressure Goal to be Achieved?

There is sufficient evidence that lower usual BP and active lowering of BP are associated with a reduction of stroke incidence. Observational studies show that decreasing 5-6 mm Hg in usual diastolic BP approximates to 35-40% lesser chances of strokes.

The exact attainable target value of BP is not absolutely clear. The decrease in BP by about 10/5 mm Hg as proposed by the PROGRESS trial has been suggested as a reasonable one for patients as per the AHA/ASA (American Heart Association/American Stroke Association) guidelines. Nevertheless, the optimal BP range and the patient's response to reduction in BP vary, when age is taken into account; hence this criterion must be considered before attempting to lower BP. Though National and International guidelines recommend aggressive BP control to <130/80 mm Hg for hypertension associated with coronary artery disease, diabetes or chronic kidney disease or <140/90 mm Hg for uncomplicated hypertension, large clinical outcome trials have observed a J-curve effect between a diastolic blood pressure of <80 mm Hg as well as a systolic blood pressure of <130 mm Hg and have cast some doubt regarding aggressive BP treatment.

Several investigators have noted that these recommendations were informed by wisdom, not facts and in majority of the clinical trials which have produced benefits from the treatment of hypertension, BP was rarely reduced to 140/90 mm Hg.

Apart from the facts and researches proposed above, it becomes difficult to decide upon the favorable target value of BP to be attained precisely and if such lesser BP values are otherwise harmless and effective. The HOT (Hypertension Optimal Treatment) trial found that however decreasing the systolic and diastolic blood pressure of hypertensive patients to 140 mm Hg and 85 mm Hg or lower, respectively was considered favorable and reduced cardiovascular complications considerably, further decrease of the systolic pressure to 120 mm Hg and diastolic pressure to 70 mm Hg added little benefit, but did not cause significant harm. An absolute target BP level and reduction are not certain and should be individualized, but benefit has been associated with an average decrease by approximately 10/5 mm Hg, and normal BP levels have been defined as <120/80 mm Hg by JNC 7. BP should be lowered gradually in patients with existing cerebrovascular disease, especially with long-standing uncontrolled hypertension.

Which Class of Antihypertensive Agent?

All the major classes of antihypertensive agents including diuretics, β-blockers, calcium-channel blockers, angiotensin-converting enzyme (ACE) inhibitors, and angiotensin receptor blockers (ARBs) seem to reduce the susceptibility to primary and recurrent stroke. The optimal drug regimen that is required to attain the recommended level of reduction is not certain as there are limited comparative studies between the different types of regimens. It has been suggested in some studies that ACE inhibitors and ARBs seem to be more effective in preventing recurrent stroke than other antihypertensive drugs; however, this has not been validated in the recent studies. The choice of specific drugs should be individualized on the basis of pharmacological properties, mechanism of action, and consideration of specific patient characteristics for which specific agents are probably indicated.

For instance, various agents may target different patient conditions like extracranial cerebrovascular occlusive disease, renal impairment, cardiac disease, and diabetes. Population with baseline blood pressure levels ≥15 to 20/10 mm Hg above the target goal value may require a multidrug therapy, and not just one agent. According to meta-analyses of randomized controlled trials, BP lowering is associated with a 30–40% reduction in stroke risk.

Reduction in risk is greater with larger reductions in BP without clear evidence of a drug class–specific treatment effect. Therefore, based on somewhat limited data, the degree of BP-lowering may be more important than the agent used.

Can Blood Pressure Lowering Result in Recurrent Stroke?

Reduction of BP in old-aged, in particular, may lead to cerebral hypoperfusion and stroke, especially in presence of focal or multifocal occlusive cerebrovascular disease. Several trials such as SHEP (Systolic Hypertension in the Elderly Program), the Syst-Eur (Systolic Hypertension in Europe) Trial, and the STOP (Swedish Trial in Old Patients with Hypertension) have shown that reducing BP considerably decreases the susceptibility to stroke and reasonable BP lowering did not lead to stroke or hypotension-related symptoms. However, individual variation in response to reduction in BP exists and this must be taken into consideration when titrating BP to a target goal in an individual patient. A majority of them sustains gradual reduction in BP, though close examination of their neurologic status is advised.

Apart from drug regimen, lifestyle modifications play a major role in lowering BP and are a reasonable part of a comprehensive antihypertensive therapy. These modifications include limiting salt intake, weight loss, consuming a diet rich in fruits and vegetables, and low-fat dairy products, routine aerobic physical exercise, and limited alcohol consumption.

CONCLUSION

Hypertension is the crucial risk factor for primary stroke. In addition, hypertension elevates the susceptibility to recurrent strokes and cardiovascular morbidity and mortality. Various studies present numerous favorable effects of reducing BP in those who are prone to ischemic stroke and at reduced risk of new or recurrent episode of stroke and other cardiovascular complications. Large-scale studies suggest beneficial effects with all classes of antihypertensive agents and choice of agent may be guided by individual patient characteristics and comorbidities. Therefore, based on somewhat limited data, the degree of BP-lowering may be more important than the agent used. The target BP levels for patients with stroke have not been delineated, but guidelines recommend aggressive BP control to <140/90 mm Hg for uncomplicated hypertension or <130/80 mm Hg for hypertension associated with coronary artery disease, diabetes or chronic kidney disease. Evidence from several studies suggest that it might be reasonable to start oral antihypertensives as soon as 24–72 hours after onset of symptoms provided there are no contraindications, but there is no definitive data to guide decisions regarding optimum time for initiating antihypertensive therapy after acute ischemic stroke.

SUGGESTED READING

1. Winstein CJ, Stein J, Arena R, et al. Guidelines for adult stroke rehabilitation and recovery: A guideline for healthcare professionals from the American Heart Association/American Stroke Association. Stroke. 2016;47(6):e98-e169.
2. Furie KL, Kasner SE, Adams RJ, et al. Guidelines for the prevention of stroke in patients with stroke or transient ischemic attack. Stroke. 2011;42(1):227-76.
3. Venkatesh Aiyagari, Philip B. Gorelick. Management of blood pressure for acute and recurrent stroke. Stroke. 2009;40(6):2251-6.
4. Castilla-Guerra L, Fernandez-Moreno Mdel C. Chronic management of hypertension after stroke: The role of ambulatory blood pressure monitoring. J Stroke. 2016;18(1):31-7.
5. Mishra NK, Patel H, Hastak SM. Comprehensive stroke care: An overview. JAPI. 2006;54:36-41.
6. Chobanian AV, Bakris GL, Black HR, et al. The Seventh Report of the Joint National Committee on Prevention, Detection, Evaluation, and Treatment of High Blood Pressure: the JNC 7 report. JAMA. 2003;289:2560-72.
7. Goldstein LB, Adams R, Alberts MJ, et al. Primary prevention of ischemic stroke: a guideline from the American Heart Association/American Stroke Association Stroke Council. Stroke. 2006;37:1583-633.
8. Castilla-Guerra L, Fernández-Moreno Mdel C. Update on the management of hypertension for secondary stroke prevention. Eur Neurol. 2012;68:1-7.

SECTION 8
Secondary Hypertension Cases

Anupam Prakash

CASE 1: Pheochromocytoma

A 40-year-old male presented with episodic headache, sweating, and palpitations for 2 years. He had been to several doctors, but no apparent abnormality was detected or found. Patient presently reported that he had become more anxious over this period and had been prescribed tablet alprazolam 0.5 mg bid, but with no benefit. The patient also informed that in recent times, the episodes had become more frequent, occurring virtually every week.

Systemic examination of the patient was normal. The patient was advised for routine blood and urine hematology and biochemistry investigations along with electrocardiogram (ECG) and chest X-ray. The patient came after 3 days with all reports being normal, but the patient was having the particular episode of headache, sweating, and palpitations. A repeat examination revealed that patient had a blood pressure of 180/110 mm Hg and was sweating profusely. ECG performed during the time showed sinus tachycardia of 128 beats per minute.

Q1. What is the likely differential diagnosis in this case?
   a. Anxiety neurosis
   b. Indolent lymphomas with type B symptoms
   c. Cardiac tachyarrhythmias
   d. Pheochromocytoma

Q2. What is the next investigation, which should be advised in this case?
   a. 24-hour ECG monitoring
   b. Electrophysiological studies
   c. Detailed psychiatric assessment
   d. 24-hour urinary vanillylmandelic acid/metanephrines

Q3. What imaging modality should be advised for this patient?
   a. Chest X-ray
   b. Abdominal Ultrasonography
   c. Abdominal CT scan
   d. Whole-body CT scan

Q4. If the abdominal CT scan in such a case is normal, but the urinary metanephrines are elevated, then what is the next step to confirm a suspected diagnosis of pheochromocytoma?
   a. Whole body CT scan
   b. MRI of the abdomen

c. MIBG scan
   d. Exploratory laparotomy

Q5. **What antihypertensive agent is preferred for control of hypertension in pheochromocytoma?**
   a. Beta-blockers
   b. Alpha-blockers
   c. Phenoxybenzamine for about a week followed by β-blocker use
   d. Calcium channel blockers

Q6. **What is the preferred modality of treatment for pheochromocytoma?**
   a. Use of anxiolytics
   b. Pharmacological management of hypertension
   c. Masterly inactivity
   d. Surgical resection of tumor

Ans. 1-d, 2-d, 3-c, 4-c, 5-c, 6-d

DISCUSSION

The differential diagnosis of episodic headache, sweating, and palpitations could include anxiety neurosis, chronic illnesses with constitutional symptoms, pheochromocytoma, or cardiac tachyarrhythmias. However, it is pertinent to note that anxiety neurosis patients usually have a stressor or trigger for anxiety episodes. At times, they could lose weight over such a long period of time, especially if the anxiety episodes are worsening as in this case. Tremors could also be noteworthy, and a detailed examination in confidence will indicate the mental state of the patient and also reveal the situations which worsen the anxiety state. Episodic symptoms could be seen with tachyarrhythmias as in paroxysmal supraventricular tachycardia. However, episodic palpitations are the main complaint and headache and sweating are usually not characteristic features. Type B symptoms associated with indolent lymphomas are usually associated with night sweats and weight loss, occasionally fever too, and these are progressive. Over a 2-year period, some lymph node groups are likely to be palpable on a systemic examination. The palpitations along with headache and sweating indicate sympathetic system activation, the episodic nature virtually indicating a release of catecholamines and documentation of severe hypertension during one such episode is a pointer toward a diagnosis of pheochromocytoma. The fact that these episodes have become more frequent over a period of time is also suggestive of a growing tumor. Patients of pheochromocytoma may have episodic hypertension or continuous hypertension, but the episodic nature of symptoms is a helpful aid to the clinician in arriving at an early diagnosis. A family history is also relevant in such a case, because pheochromocytomas can occur as part of multiple endocrine neoplasia type 2 (MEN2), von Hippel–Lindau syndrome, and neurofibromatosis type 1.

At times, thyrotoxicosis patients may have hypertension, sweating, and palpitations. However, the hypertension is never severe, and invariably the episodic nature of symptoms is missing. Resting tachycardia is an important feature of thyrotoxicosis patients. Testing for thyroid function tests can easily help in establishing the diagnosis.

If one were to investigate such a case, as already stated, an ordinary interaction with the patient in confidence is usually sufficient to reveal a diagnosis of anxiety neurosis to an observant clinician. However, a detailed psychiatric assessment would always come in handy, if required. A 24-hour ECG recording or electrophysiologic studies would be appropriate, if one was suspecting tachyarrhythmias in this patient. However, as already discussed, it would be prudent to investigate this case for 24-hour urinary vanillylmandelic acid or metanephrine levels. Presence of high levels of urinary concentrations indicates a greater production from the adrenal tumor (87.5% sensitivity and 99.7% specificity for pheochromocytoma).

Therefore, in such a scenario, the next line of investigation is to visualize the tumor in the adrenals so as to localize the pheochromocytoma. Pheochromocytoma is a benign tumor, but can be malignant in up to 10% of the cases. In 10% of the cases, bilateral pheochromocytoma may be present, while in 10% of the cases, extra-adrenal pheochromocytomas (paragangliomas) may be observed. Computed tomography (CT) scan of the abdomen is the preferred imaging modality to localize the adrenal tumor masses, with a sensitivity of 85–95% with a spatial resolution of 1 cm or greater. Magnetic resonance imaging (MRI) is preferred in children and pregnant and lactating women, wherein it has a reported sensitivity of 100% in detecting pheochromocytomas. However, at times the imaging modalities may not show a tumor, despite biochemical confirmation in form of elevated metanephrines. In such cases, it is wise to get Iodine-131 metaiodobenzylguanidine (131I-MIBG) scintigraphy done to localize the pheochromocytoma. Some doctors prefer to get it done as a routine before taking an invasive procedure, i.e., before taking the patient for surgery.

Isolated β-blocker use to control hypertension can result in unopposed alpha stimulation resulting in hypertensive crisis and its serious consequences. Therefore, it is recommended to initiate α-blockade with phenoxybenzamine and after 7–10 days noncardioselective β-blocker agent (propranolol) is added, following which subject should be taken up for surgical resection of the tumor.

Surgery offers cure from not only the symptoms, but from hypertension as well. Usually the tumor is >3 cm, when the symptoms are so much, as in this case. Localizing the tumor is also important because of determining the location and also to see if bilateral tumors are present. Moreover, surgery is helpful because 10% cases may turn out to be malignant. It is noteworthy that pheochromocytoma is a secondary cause of hypertension and surgical resection of the tumor is cures hypertension.

CASE 2: Conn Syndrome

A 50-year-male presented with history of headache and generalized muscle weakness for 6–8 months, for which he showed to a doctor, and was diagnosed to be hypertensive 1 year back (BP 140/100 mm Hg). He was initially started on cilnidipine 10 mg and hydrochlorothiazide 12.5 mg daily, which was doubled at 6 weeks. His symptoms of headache and weakness persisted. At 3 months, losartan 100 mg once daily was added, but symptoms did not improve. His blood pressure on the last visit was 136/96 mm Hg in both upper arms, and has remained between 130–140 systolic and 90–100 mm Hg diastolic in the last 6 months. Body mass index (BMI) was 21 kg/m². Systemic examination was normal, there was no pedal edema or signs of heart failure.

Routine blood hematology was normal and blood biochemistry revealed normal serum lipid profile and liver function tests, blood urea: 25 mg/dL, serum creatinine: 0.6 mg/dL, serum sodium: 148 mEq/L, and serum potassium: 3.3 mEq/L. ECG and chest X-ray were normal.

Q1. What is this hypertension referred to as?
a. White-coat hypertension
b. Resistant hypertension
c. Secondary hypertension
d. Pseudoresistance hypertension

Q2. Which of the following is a cause of secondary hypertension?
a. Pheochromocytoma
b. Conn's syndrome
c. Cushing's syndrome
d. All of the above

Q3. Pseudoresistance (false resistant hypertension) can be because of:
A. Inadequate doses of antihypertensive drugs
B. Inappropriate antihypertensive combinations
C. Poor adherence to desired lifestyle (viz. dietary sodium restriction)
D. All of the above

Q4. What is the likely etiology in the above case?
a. Cushing's syndrome
b. Conn's syndrome
c. Pheochromocytoma
d. Essential hypertension

Q5. What is the most common cause of primary hyperaldosteronism?
a. Bilateral idiopathic adrenal hyperplasia
b. Adrenal adenoma
c. Adrenocortical carcinoma
d. Ectopic aldosterone-producing adenoma or carcinoma

Q6. Complication of untreated hyperaldosteronism includes:
a. Cerebrovascular disease or Stroke
b. Cardiovascular disease
c. Kidney disease
d. All of the above

Q7. Diastolic hypertension without edema is a feature of:
a. Cushing's syndrome
b. Primary hyperaldosteronism
c. Pheochromocytoma
d. Essential hypertension

Ans. 1-b, 2-d, 3-d, 4-b, 5-a, 6-d, 7-b

DISCUSSION

The present case is likely to be a case of secondary hypertension, but definitely fulfills the criteria for resistant hypertension. Resistant hypertension is the inability to control blood pressure (<140/90 mm Hg) with the use of three classes of drugs, in maximal or near maximal doses, of which one is a thiazide diuretic.

Causes contributing to secondary hypertension are a major cause of resistant hypertension. Pheochromocytoma, Conn's syndrome (better known as primary hyperaldosteronism) and Cushing's syndrome are all secondary causes of hypertension, having their origin from the adrenal gland.

At times, pseudoresistance can be seen and the important causes for pseudoresistance are given in **Box 1**.

Box 1: Causes of false resistant hypertension or pseudoresistance.
- Lack of adherence to lifestyle advice including dietary restriction of sodium
- Poor monitoring of blood pressure
- White-coat resistant hypertension
- Noncompliance with antihypertensive medications:
  ○ Side effects of antihypertensive medications
  ○ Complicated dosing regimens
  ○ Deficiency in patient education
  ○ High costs of drugs
  ○ Cuff-related artifacts
  ○ Psychiatric issues
  ○ Poor cognition in elderly
- Physician-related factors:
  ○ Poor blood pressure measuring technique
  ○ Clinical inertia
  ○ Inadequate doses of antihypertensive drugs/inappropriate dosing pattern
  ○ Using wrong combination of antihypertensive agents
  ○ Poor information, education and communication (IEC) related issues

The likely diagnosis in this case of refractory hypertension is likely to be primary hyperaldosteronism, also referred to as Conn's syndrome. The suggestion to this diagnosis comes from the history of generalized muscle weakness reported by this patient from the very beginning of the illness, coupled with a primarily diastolic hypertension, and supported by the presence of high serum sodium levels and hypokalemia. Aldosterone induces the renal reabsorption of sodium at the distal convoluted tubule and the medullary collecting duct. It acts on the principal cells, increasing activity of the basolateral sodium-potassium ATPase and apical epithelial sodium channels (ENaC), as well as renal outer medullary K^+ (ROMK) channels potassium channels (ROMK) causing increased sodium reabsorption and enhancing the secretion of potassium and hydrogen ions, causing hypernatremia, hypokalemia, and alkalosis.

Further screening test includes a plasma aldosterone to plasma renin activity ratio which would be raised. The sodium retention and the plasma volume expansion secondary to hyperaldosteronism results in increased glomerular filtration rate and diminished renin release from the juxtaglomerular apparatus. This decrease in renin release does not result in a reduction of aldosterone levels in primary hyperaldosteronism. Therefore, the plasma aldosterone to plasma renin activity will be raised. However, in cases of secondary hyperaldosteronism, both plasma renin activity and plasma aldosterone levels are raised.

Confirmatory tests include 24-hour urinary aldosterone excretion test or a salt loading test. The type of hyperaldosteronism can be determined by the postural stimulation test or the furosemide stimulation test or diurnal rhythm of aldosterone.

Primary hyperaldosteronism can constitute 5–15% of the cases of hypertension, though earlier it was believed that it contributed to <1% of the hypertension cases. As already stated, recognizing this entity requires a high degree of suspicion, which is essential since the management varies with its diagnosis and the likely cause of primary hyperaldosteronism.

Bilateral idiopathic adrenal hyperplasia is the most common cause of primary hyperaldosteronism (almost two-thirds of the cases) followed by adrenal adenomas (one-third of the cases). The latter condition was described by Conn originally, when he described an adrenal adenoma, which came to be known as Conn's tumor and this condition of primary hyperaldosteronism was given the name of Conn's syndrome. Less commonly (<1% cases), primary hyperaldosteronism is caused by adrenal adenocarcinoma, familial forms of primary aldosteronism, or ectopic secretion of aldosterone.

A high-resolution thin sliced (2–2.5 mm) adrenal CT scan with contrast is helpful in localizing the pathology. In cases, where the biochemical evidence of hyperaldosteronism exists but the tumor is not localized, adrenal venous sampling may be utilized. Also in cases, where there is a nonfunctioning adenoma and bilateral adrenal hyperplasia, adrenal venous sampling is helpful. Dexamethasone suppression test is of value only in cases of possible familial aldosteronism.

Pharmacological therapy includes use of mineralocorticoid antagonists like spironolactone and eplerenone. Calcium channel blockers are additionally helpful apart from dietary sodium restriction. Surgery (adrenalectomy) offers permanent cure in cases of aldosteronoma and other lateralizable causes of hyperaldosteronism.

CASE 3: Thyrotoxicosis with Hypertension

A 38-year-old female presented with progressive weight gain and depressed mood over a period of 2–3 years. Family history, dietary history, and past medical history were noncontributory. Patient was not taking any medicines (allopathic or indigenous) or oral contraceptive pills. Patient had two children aged 10 years and 15 years of age and menstrual history was normal.

Examination revealed blood pressure of 160/102 mm Hg in both arms, plethoric face, predominantly truncal obesity, and wide violaceous striae on the abdomen. Bilateral pitting pedal edema was present. Neurological system examination revealed that patient was requiring support in getting up from the squatting position; however, the reflexes were all normal. Investigations revealed impaired glucose tolerance state.

Q1. What is the likely diagnosis in this case?
   a. Myxedema
   b. Depression
   c. Polycystic ovarian disease
   d. Cushing's syndrome

Q2. What investigation should be advised to this patient?
   a. 24-hour urinary cortisol estimation
   b. Serum ACTH levels
   c. CT adrenals
   d. Serum aldosterone levels

Q3. Which one of the following could be a possible cause of Cushing's syndrome in this case?
   a. Adrenal tumor
   b. Oral contraceptive use
   c. Exogenous administration of steroids
   d. All of the above

Q4. Which of the following is a feature of Nelson's syndrome?
   a. Skin pigmentation
   b. Visual field defects
   c. Amenorrhea
   d. All of the above

Q5. Elevated cortisol levels on inferior petrosal vein sampling indicate:
   a. Adrenal cause of Cushing's syndrome
   b. Pituitary cause of Cushing's syndrome
   c. Iatrogenic Cushing's syndrome
   d. Ectopic ACTH production

Ans. 1-d, 2-a, 3-a, 4-d, 5-b

DISCUSSION

Depression, hypothyroidism, polycystic ovarian disease, and oral contraceptive use (though patient denies history of use of contraceptives in this case) can all present with mood disturbance (depression), weight gain, severe hypertension, and glucose intolerance. However, menstrual disturbances are highly likely in the former three disease conditions. Moreover, the pattern of weight gain with predilection toward the trunk and presence of wide violaceous striae and plethoric facies is a pointer toward Cushing's syndrome. Presence of proximal myopathy again is indicative of an endocrine or metabolic cause. Although myxedema can also have proximal myopathy, but pedal edema is usually nonpitting and tendon reflexes may be diminished/sluggish and characteristically ankle jerks may be hung-up (prolonged relaxation time).

Investigations in such a case are aimed at confirming the diagnosis of Cushing's syndrome and then aimed at identifying its etiology. Cushing's syndrome is a state of glucocorticoid excess, and is diagnosed by the elevated cortisol levels in blood, urine or saliva. Importantly, failure of suppression of the serum cortisol levels, after administering supraphysiological doses of dexamethasone, can be utilized in the form of overnight or 48-hour dexamethasone suppression test (1 mg dexamethasone at midnight followed by serum cortisol assessment at 8 AM or 0.5 mg dexamethasone 6 hourly for 2 days followed by serum cortisol assessment at 8 AM, respectively). Serum cortisol levels >1.8 µg/dL (normal value <5 µg/dL) or 24-hour urinary cortisol >100 µg are considered high (normal value <90 µg or 830 nmol/24 h; values >300 µg or 830 nmol/24 h are diagnostic of Cushing's syndrome). Midnight salivary cortisol can also be assessed, but is not yet available in India. Also, obesity, chronic illness, chronic alcoholism, and depression can give false-positive results (pseudo-Cushing's syndrome) on the 1 mg-dexamethasone suppression test or slightly high values on the 24-hour urinary free cortisol method.

Therefore, 24-hour urinary cortisol or the high-dose/overnight dexamethasone suppression tests can be used as screening test and the low-dose (48-hour) dexamethasone test is used as a confirmatory test. None of these tests is >95% sensitive, and hence it is considered that at least two of these tests should be positive for diagnosing Cushing's syndrome. One suggested approach is that the 48-hour dexamethasone suppression test can be combined with the corticotropin-releasing hormone (CRH) stimulation test, in which 2 hours after the last dexamethasone dose, 1 µg/kg CRH is administered intravenously, and plasma cortisol is administered 15 minutes after the injection. A plasma cortisol level >1.4 µg/L (40 nmol/L) is considered positive for Cushing's syndrome. This combination test is considered to be 100% sensitive and specific for Cushing's syndrome. Another alternative approach is to test the midnight serum cortisol, and a value <7.5 µg/dL (207 nmol/L) is strongly suggestive of pseudo-Cushing's syndrome.

The next step is to find the etiology of Cushing's syndrome. The common causes of Cushing's syndrome are enumerated in **Box 1**. Since the mechanisms are classified as adrenocorticotropic hormone (ACTH) independent and ACTH dependent, the first investigation is to get the serum ACTH levels. If the serum ACTH levels are undetectable (<10 pg/mL), it indicates an adrenal oversecretion of cortisol, wherein a CT of the adrenals should be obtained to identify the cause. In case, the ACTH levels are raised or normal, it is indicative of a pituitary cause or ectopic production of ACTH/CRH. A contrast-enhanced MRI of the pituitary can help locate an ACTH producing microadenoma. However, in the absence of a distinct pituitary lesion, inferior petrosal vein sampling is recommended, and a higher value in the inferior petrosal vein which drains the pituitary compared to any peripheral vein is suggestive of a pituitary adenoma. If there is no difference, it indicates an ectopic ACTH source which will need to be investigated upon by performing a CT of the chest and abdomen. Cushing's disease is the term specifically given to pituitary adenomas (usually microadenomas), which result in Cushing's syndrome. Characteristically ACTH secreting microadenomas result in bilateral adrenal hyperplasia and features of Cushing's syndrome.

The treatment of Cushing's syndrome is resection of the adrenal tumor or in cases of Cushing's disease transsphenoidal removal of the pituitary tumor. In cases of recurrence, pituitary irradiation can induce remission of disease in over half of the patients. Patients who are not cured may require total bilateral adrenalectomy for symptom alleviation. In patients of Cushing's disease, undergoing bilateral adrenalectomy, pigmentation may be observed because of excessive ACTH secretion, and headache, visual disturbances, or menstrual abnormalities may be witnessed because of pressure symptoms on the adjoining structures in the pituitary fossa. This is known as Nelson's syndrome.

Cushing's syndrome resulting from exogenous administration of steroids results in undetectable serum ACTH and cortisol levels, and hence, a historical detailed evaluation is a must to elicit this history.

> **Box 1: Etiology of Cushing's syndrome.**
> - *ACTH-dependent:*
>   - Pituitary adenoma
>   - Ectopic ACTH production
>   - Ectopic CRH production
> - *ACTH-independent:*
>   - Adrenal adenoma
>   - Adrenal carcinoma
>   - Primary adrenal hyperplasia
> - Exogenous administration of glucocorticoids

(ACTH: adrenocorticotropic hormone; CRH: corticotropin-releasing hormone)

CASE 4: Hypothyroidism with Hypertension

A 55-year-old female presented with complaints of tremors of hands, prominence of both eyes, weight loss, palpitations, and heat intolerance for the last 6 months. Examination revealed a thin-built anxious looking lady, with bilateral proptosis, fine tremors of hands, diffuse goiter, tachycardia of 120 beats per minute, blood pressure of 160/80 mm Hg, and brisk bilateral deep tendon reflexes.

Q1. What is the likely diagnosis?
   a. Anxiety neurosis
   b. Pheochromocytoma
   c. Thyrotoxicosis
   d. Carcinoid syndrome

Q2. Which of the following conditions is associated with isolated systolic hypertension?
   a. Aortic regurgitation
   b. Elderly individuals
   c. Thyrotoxicosis
   d. All of the above

Q3. Which of the following causes of hyperthyroidism is not associated with increased radioactive iodine uptake?
   a. Toxic multinodular goiter
   b. Iodide-induced hyperthyroidism
   c. Graves' disease
   d. Toxic adenoma

Q4. Which of the following entities causes thyrotoxicosis without hyperthyroidism?
   a. Subacute thyroiditis
   b. Postpartum thyroiditis
   c. Thyrotoxicosis factitia
   d. All of the above

Q5. Which of the following criteria is NOT a part of the Graves' disease triad?
   a. Diffuse toxic goiter
   b. Proximal myopathy
   c. Infiltrative dermopathy
   d. Infiltrative ophthalmopathy

Ans. 1-c, 2-d, 3-b, 4-d, 5-b

DISCUSSION

The patient has classical symptoms suggestive of thyrotoxicosis. Other characteristic features which may be seen in other cases of thyrotoxicosis include weight loss despite a good appetite, increased sweating leading to a warm moist skin, increased gastrointestinal motility, atrial tachyarrhythmias like atrial fibrillation, and a thyroid bruit. The common causes of thyrotoxicosis are enlisted in **Box 1**.

The diagnosis of thyrotoxicosis is made by excess of T3 and/or T4 levels in the blood. This is invariably associated with low serum thyroid-stimulating hormone (TSH) levels. Usually, T4 levels are high associated with low TSH levels, except in occasional cases of T3 toxicosis, wherein T3 levels are elevated and TSH levels are low, while T4 levels are normal. The most common cause of thyrotoxicosis is Graves' disease, which has the characteristic triad of diffuse goiter, infiltrative ophthalmopathy and infiltrative dermopathy. Coeliac disease, gastric achlorhydria, pernicious anemia, and myasthenia gravis may be present as other autoimmune diseases. All causes of hyperthyroidism have an increased radioactive iodine uptake except for iodide-induced hyperthyroidism. Thyroid scan in Graves' disease shows a uniform tracer distribution, while patchy distribution is seen in toxic multinodular goiter, and unifocal activity corresponding to a nodule with suppression of the rest of the thyroid gland suggests a toxic adenoma.

Methimazole, carbimazole, and propylthiouracil are the agents of choice for medical management, and act by inhibiting thyroid hormone synthesis. Propylthiouracil also inhibits extrathyroidal conversion of T4 to T3. Propylthiouracil use is reserved for first trimester of pregnancy, in patients with life-threatening thyrotoxicosis or thyroid storm, and in patients experiencing adverse effects of methimazole (except agranulocytosis).

Beta-blocker agents relieve the adrenergic symptoms of palpitations, tremors and anxiety, apart from controlling the blood pressure, and propranolol also blocks the peripheral conversion of T4 to T3.

Box 1: Common causes of thyrotoxicosis.

- *Associated with hyperthyroidism:*
  - Graves' disease
  - Toxic multinodular goiter
  - Toxic adenoma
  - Iodide-induced hyperthyroidism
  - Trophoblastic tumor
  - Increased thyroid-stimulating hormone (TSH) secretion
- *Not associated with hyperthyroidism:*
  - Thyrotoxicosis factitia
  - Subacute thyroiditis
  - Post-partum thyroiditis
  - Chronic thyroiditis with transient toxicosis
  - Ectopic thyroid tissue

Radioactive iodine ablation is curative in 90–95% of patients, but should not be performed in pregnant patients and patients should also not conceive for at least 6 months after ablation.

Surgery (bilateral subtotal thyroidectomy) can be offered to patients with very large goiter causing compressive symptoms, or patients with significant eye disease or those intolerant to antithyroid drugs.

CASE 5: Cushing's with Hypertension

A 45-year-old female presented with lethargy, listlessness, daytime somnolence, decreased appetite, weight gain, and menorrhagia over the last 6 months. She also complained of cold intolerance during the winter season which just got over. Examination revealed morbid obesity, dry coarse skin, hoarse voice, bilateral nonpitting pedal edema, diminished deep tendon reflexes, and a blood pressure of 130/100 mm Hg in both arms.

Q1. What is the likely clinical diagnosis?
   a. Cushing's syndrome
   b. Hypothyroidism
   c. Pickwickian syndrome
   d. Polycystic ovarian syndrome

Q2. What investigation should be ordered to confirm the diagnosis?
   a. Serum TSH, T3, and T4 levels
   b. Thyroid scan
   c. Serum LH levels
   d. Serum cortisol levels

Q3. Isolated diastolic hypertension is a feature of:
   a. Hypothyroidism
   b. Primary hyperaldosteronism
   c. Hyperparathyroidism
   d. All of the above

Q4. Which drug can be used for treatment of hypertension in hypothyroidism?
   a. Angiotensin-converting enzyme (ACE) inhibitors
   b. Calcium channel blockers
   c. Thiazide diuretics
   d. All of the above

Q5. Which test should be used to monitor the euthyroid status in hypothyroidism?
   a. Serum Free T3
   b. Serum Free T4
   c. Serum TSH
   d. Anti-TPO antibodies

Ans. 1-b, 2-a, 3-d, 4-d, 5-c

■ DISCUSSION

This patient has characteristic features of hypothyroidism, and has presented with an elevated diastolic blood pressure. In hypothyroidism, all vital signs could be on the lower side with bradycardia, low normal blood pressure, and low body temperature. However, this patient has a high diastolic blood pressure, and warrants treatment. Hypertension is not a feature of hypothyroidism and the relation is seemingly not a direct one. However, hypothyroidism, especially severe hypothyroidism can be related to accelerated atherosclerosis. Endothelial dysfunction and increased peripheral vascular resistance are also observed in hypothyroidism. Although a reduced pulse rate and reduced cardiac output in hypothyroidism suggest lower sympathetic activity, but direct measurements suggest that sympathetic activity is increased in hypothyroidism. Overt hypothyroidism is also known to be associated with atherogenic dyslipidemia, and elevated carotid intima media thickness. Besides, subclinical hypothyroidism is an accepted independent risk factor for coronary heart disease. Therefore, several mechanisms play a role in causation of hypertension in patients with hypothyroidism. Notably, although hypertension associated with hypothyroidism can be said to be secondary hypertension, but this secondary hypertension is somewhat unique, in the sense that it is not completely remediable with the control of the cause, i.e., hypothyroidism in the present case. Therefore, even when the patient of hypothyroidism becomes euthyroid, the hypertension does not resolve completely, but requires antihypertensive medications to keep the blood pressure within normal limits. This is unlike the other conditions causing secondary hypertension viz. pheochromocytoma, Conn's syndrome, Cushing's syndrome, hyperthyroidism, etc., where resection of the tumor/lesion actually remits hypertension completely, and there is no need for antihypertensive agents in most of the cases.

The diagnosis of overt primary hypothyroidism is confirmed biochemically by the presence of an elevated serum TSH level associated with low serum levels of thyroid hormones (T3 and T4). Subclinical hypothyroidism is diagnosed by an elevated serum TSH level associated with normal levels of thyroid hormones. Follow-up of euthyroid status can be done by getting serum TSH levels. The aim is to maintain serum TSH levels between 2 µU/mL and 3 µU/mL. Normal levels of serum TSH are in the range of 0.5–4.5 µU/mL, serum T3: 80–220 ng/dL, and serum T4: 4.5–12.5 µg/dL.

In overt hypothyroidism patients, oral thyroxine replacement is the treatment of choice (1.6–1.7 µg/kg lean body weight). Subclinical hypothyroidism also needs to be treated if the serum TSH levels are above 12 µU/mL. If the serum TSH levels are between 8 µU/mL and 12 µU/mL then symptomatic cases may need to be treated with thyroxine viz. infertility, menstrual disturbances, dyslipidemia, or weight gain attributable to hypothyroidism.

There is no preferential choice of antihypertensive medications for treatment of hypertension in hypothyroidism. However, there could be some concern with β-blockers since they are known to inhibit the peripheral conversion of T4 to T3. However, of greater concern could be the delayed metabolism in overt hypothyroid subjects till the time they become euthyroid. All five groups of antihypertensive drugs can be employed for control of blood pressure in hypothyroid subjects, i.e., ACE inhibitors or angiotensin receptor blockers, calcium channel blockers, α-blockers, β-blockers, and diuretics.

SUGGESTED READINGS

1. Thakur BB, Thakur S. Resistant Hypertension. In: Munjal YP (Ed). API Textbook of Medicine, 10th edition India: Association of Physicians of India; 2015. pp. 930-4.
2. Bhatia E, Bhatia V. Disorders of adrenal glands. In: Munjal YP (Ed). API Textbook of Medicine, 10th edition. India: Association of Physicians of India; 2015. pp. 610-20.
3. Tandon N, Raizada N. Disorders of thyroid glands. In: Munjal YP (Ed). API Textbook of Medicine, 10th edition. India: Association of Physicians of India; 2015. pp. 592-605.
4. Kirk LF Jr, Hash RB, Katner HP, et al. Cushing's disease: clinical manifestations and diagnostic evaluation. Am Fam Physician. 2000;62:1119-27.

SECTION 9
Cardiac Effects

Gurpreet S Wander

CASE 1: Hypertension and Heart Failure with a Preserved Ejection Fraction

A 55-year-old man admitted to hospital with worsening dyspnea from New York Heart Association (NYHA) Class II to NYHA Class III over past 6 months. He has been known hypertensive since past 10 years, but was poorly compliant with medications. He denies exertional chest pain. He sleeps on two pillows and has some mild ankle edema.

On examination, the heart rate was 102 beats/min, blood pressure was 150/90 mm Hg, and respiratory rate was 22 breaths/min. Bilateral pedal edema was present. Respiratory system revealed bilateral basal crepitations. Cardiovascular examination was essentially normal.

An electrocardiogram did not demonstrate ischemic changes and was within normal limits.

Chest X-ray was suggestive of pulmonary venous hypertension (PVH) with bilateral blunting of costophrenic (CP) angles.

Baseline echocardiography showed mild left ventricular hypertrophy (LVH), with septal and posterior wall thickness of 12 mm and an LV end-diastolic dimension of 4.5 cm, with LV ejection fraction (LVEF) of 60%. Mitral inflow pattern showed an E:A ratio of 1.8 that changed with Valsalva to an impaired relaxed pattern with a septal annular E' velocity of 7.2 cm/s. Her resting pulmonary artery systolic pressure (PASP) was 55 mm Hg.

Q1. Which of the following statements is incorrect?
   a. The majority of elderly patients with heart failure have reduced LVEF
   b. Systolic hypertension has the highest population attributable risk for the development of heart failure
   c. Morbidity and mortality are similar in patients with heart failure with reduced and preserved ejection fraction (HFrEF and HFpEF)
   d. Five-year mortality rate in patients with newly diagnosed heart failure is 50% or higher

Q2. Treatment with which of the following class of drugs provides mortality benefit in patients with HFpEF?
   a. Angiotensin-converting enzyme (ACE) inhibitor
   b. Mineralocorticoid receptor antagonist
   c. Beta-blockers
   d. None of above

Q3. Most common rhythm abnormality seen in heart failure with normal ejection fraction (HFnEF) is:
   a. Ventricular premature contractions
   b. Ventricular tachycardia
   c. Atrial fibrillation
   d. Multifocal atrial tachycardia

Q4. Which of the following statements is correct?
   a. Brain natriuretic peptide (BNP) levels in HFnEF are lower than in HFrEF
   b. All patients with HFnEF show left ventricular hypertrophy on echocardiogram
   c. HFnEF is more common in males than in females
   d. Takotsubo cardiomyopathy is a form of HFnEF

Ans. 1-a, 2-d, 3-c, 4-a

DISCUSSION

Patients with heart failure can be categorized into three, as the ones with:
- Heart failure with a reduced ejection fraction (HFrEF).
- Heart failure with a preserved ejection fraction (HFpEF).
- Heart failure with mid-range ejection fraction (HFmrEF).

The patients who are considered to have "recovered" HFrEF are those who previously had an ejection fraction (EF) <40% but with EF increased in them with therapy for heart failure.

Ventricular diastolic dysfunction, i.e., impaired relaxation and increased diastolic stiffness, present at rest or caused by stress (due to exercise, hypertension, or tachycardia), is considered to be a central perturbation in HFpEF. Abnormal diastolic function can occur with normal/abnormal systolic function or in the presence/absence of a clinical syndrome of heart failure. Diastolic dysfunction refers to abnormal LV performance; whereas HFpEF refers to a clinical syndrome of heart failure.

Though EF is normal at rest, it does not increase appropriately with stress, and other measures of systolic function are abnormal.

Epidemiology and Natural History

Among the patients with heart failure, 50% are found to have a preserved EF, and there is an increase in this proportion over time. Compared with those with a reduced EF, patients with preserved EF are older and more likely to be female. The most common antecedent disease leading to HFpEF is systolic hypertension, which is present in >85% of patients. Obesity is seen in 30–50%, diabetes in 20–30%, and atrial fibrillation in up to 20–30% of patients.

Rates of hospitalization and death in the patients with HFpEF are close to the patients with HFrEF. In patients who have HFpEF, there is a devastating 5-year mortality rate (reaching 60%) as well as morbidity (6-month hospitalization rate being 50%). Most (>70%) of the deaths in patients with HFpEF are cardiovascular in nature, with 20% due to heart failure and 35% due to sudden death. This distribution of modes of cardiovascular death is similar to that for HFrEF. The incidence of noncardiovascular deaths is significantly higher for HFpEF (30%) than for HFrEF (15%), reflecting the higher age and increased comorbidity in patients with HFpEF.

Pathophysiology

Common findings include arterial stiffening, endothelial dysfunction, and enhanced ventricular systolic stiffness; these may cause increased sensitivity to changes in load. This sensitivity presents as rapid-onset pulmonary edema with increase in load and excessive hypotension with decrease in load.

Diagnosis and Evaluation (Flowchart 1)

Signs and symptoms of heart failure are nonspecific, and therefore require a high index of suspicion for heart failure among patients with risk factors. Alternative or contributing diagnoses must also be considered.

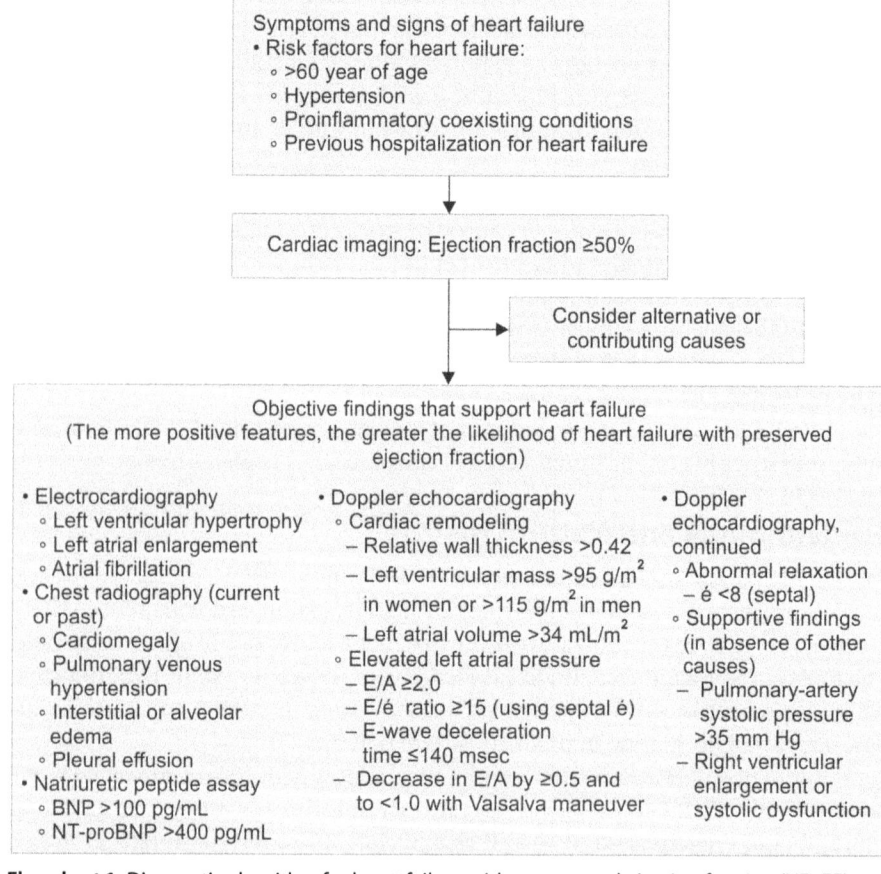

Flowchart 1: Diagnostic algorithm for heart failure with a preserved ejection fraction (HFpEF).

The size of the left ventricular cavity is usually normal. Evidence of LVH is common but absent in many patients. Evidence of diastolic dysfunction on Doppler echocardiography (which includes slowed ventricular relaxation and enhanced diastolic stiffness or increased left atrial pressure) is a common finding. Nevertheless, diastolic dysfunction may be noted among patients who are not having heart failure and absent among patients who received aggressive treatment for heart failure or in patients having predominantly exertional symptoms. Usually, the left atrium is enlarged. Pulmonary artery systolic pressure (PASP) is usually increased (>35 mm Hg). Right ventricular systolic dysfunction, usually in association with atrial fibrillation, is present in 20-30% patients. The atrial remodeling can result in annular dilatation as well as functional mitral and tricuspid regurgitation, however primary valvular disease should be excluded.

As compared to the patients with HFrEF, patients with HFpEF have lower ventricular wall stress and therefore lower circulating levels of natriuretic peptides. On an average, brain natriuretic peptide (BNP) value in patients with HFpEF who present with acute decompensation is 100–500 pg/mL, as compared to 500–1,500 pg/mL among patients who have HFrEF. There may be normal levels of natriuretic peptides in nearly 30% patients with HFpEF, specifically among obese patients or those patients who have purely exertional symptoms. The higher the level of natriuretic peptide, the greater the possibility of patient having heart failure. But, in some advanced age patients or those with atrial fibrillation without heart failure, levels of natriuretic peptide are comparable to those of patients with HF.

Treatment (Flowchart 2)

In patients with HFpEF, improvement in outcomes has not been shown by any therapy. Existing therapy consists of the following:
- Relief of volume overload
- Treatment of coexisting conditions
- Other strategies that may lead to enhanced exercise tolerance or reduction of symptoms
- Strategies for management of chronic disease and prevention of hospitalizations.

Trials of Therapies to Improve Outcomes

In individual trials or in a meta-analysis, randomized trials of angiotensin antagonists [i.e., angiotensin-converting enzyme (ACE) inhibitors or angiotensin II receptor blocker (ARB)] which included patients with HFpEF did not show significant effects of these agents on composite end points of all-cause or cardiovascular mortality as well as hospitalizations for heart failure.

The mineralocorticoid-receptor antagonist spironolactone did not reduce rates of the primary composite outcome of death from cardiovascular causes, aborted cardiac arrest, or hospitalization for heart failure in these patients.

The rate of hospitalization for heart failure was decreased by spironolactone. Spironolactone reduced the rate of hospitalization for heart failure but not the rate of death from any cause or hospitalization for any cause, and it increased the rate of renal dysfunction and hyperkalemia.

In patients who have heart failure and a preserved EF, the effect of beta-blockers has not been assessed in a sufficiently powered study. The data available are limited and conflicting.

Therefore, for the treatment of patients with HFpEF, using angiotensin antagonists and beta-blockers should be restricted to those patients who have optional indications for their usage. It is still a controversy to use spironolactone in patients with HFpEF.

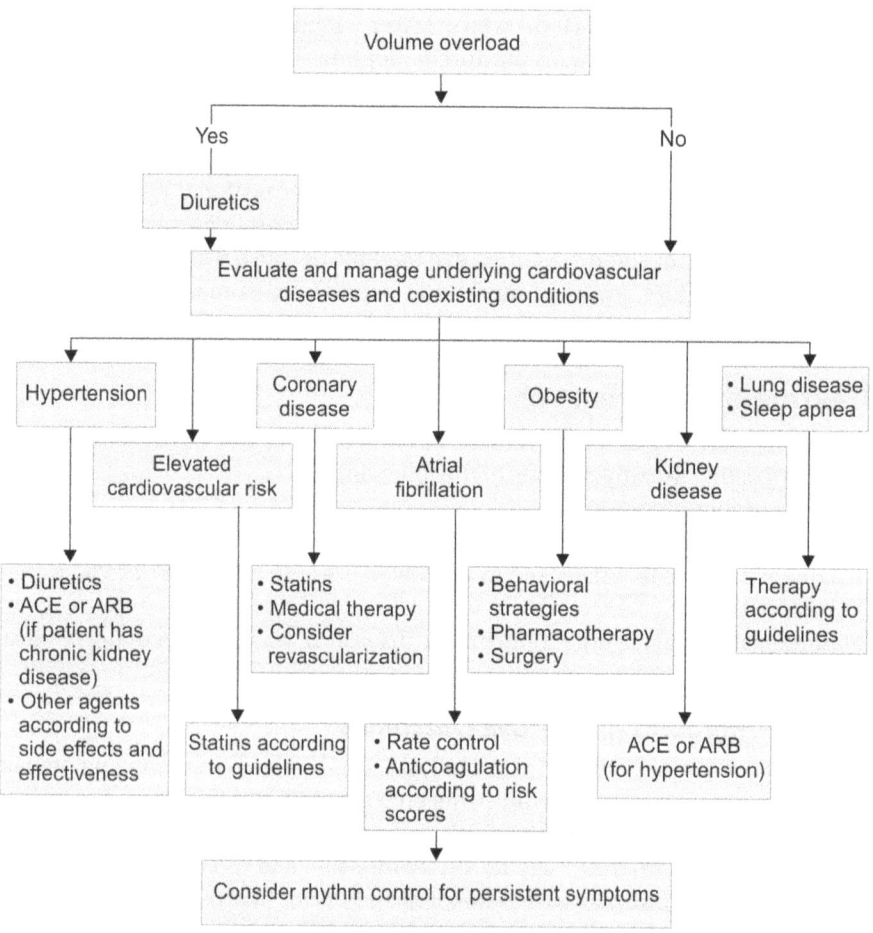

(ACE: angiotensin-converting enzyme; ARB: angiotensin II receptor blocker)

Flowchart 2: Algorithm for management of patients with heart failure with normal ejection fraction (HFnEF).

KEY POINTS
- Among patients with signs and symptoms of heart failure but a preserved EF, electrocardiography, echocardiography, chest radiography, and measurement of levels of natriuretic peptide should be used for confirmation of objective evidence of abnormal cardiac structure as well as function.
- Natriuretic peptide levels may be normal in patients who have heart failure with a preserved EF, particularly in obese patients or those with symptoms only on exertion.
- The medications that were shown to improve outcomes in patients with HFrEF have not been shown to provide benefit in those with HFpEF.
- HFpEF treatment should comprise of treatment for coexisting cardiovascular and noncardiovascular conditions, diuretics for volume overload, education related to self-care, aerobic exercise training for enhancing exercise tolerance, and disease management programs in patients who have refractory symptoms or repeated hospitalizations for heart failure.

SUGGESTED READING
1. Ponikowski P, Voors AA, Anker SD, et al. 2016 ESC Guidelines for the diagnosis and treatment of acute and chronic heart failure: The Task Force for the diagnosis and treatment of acute and chronic heart failure of the European Society of Cardiology (ESC) Developed with the special contribution of the Heart Failure Association (HFA) of the ESC. Eur Heart J. 2016;37(27):2129-200.
2. Redfield MM. Heart failure with preserved ejection fraction. N Engl J Med. 2016;375(19): 1868-77.

CASE 2: Hypertension and Coronary Artery Disease

A 65-year-old hypertensive female came to OPD with complaints of anginal chest discomfort over past 6 months. Her medications included tablet amlodipine 5 mg twice a day and tablet hydrochlorothiazide 12.5 mg once daily.

On examination, her heart rate was 96 beats/min, blood pressure was 160/100 mm Hg, and respiratory rate was 14 breaths/min. Cardiovascular (CV) examination was essentially normal with no S_3 or S_4.

An electrocardiogram (ECG) demonstrated T-wave inversion in V_1–V_6. Baseline echocardiography showed normal left ventricular (LV) systolic and diastolic function and no regional wall motion abnormalities.

Q1. Which of the following is drug of choice for hypertension in a person with coronary artery disease (CAD) and angina?
   a. Alpha-blocker
   b. Beta-blocker
   c. Calcium channel blocker (CCB)
   d. Angiotensin II receptor blocker (ARB)

Q2. The association of hypertension and coronary heart disease is a frequent one. Which of the following pathophysiologic mechanisms link both diseases?
   a. Endothelial dysfunction
   b. Renin–angiotensin–aldosterone system (RAAS) activation
   c. Increased sympathetic drive
   d. All of the above

Q3. Which of the following antianginal drugs has no hemodynamic effect?
   a. Metoprolol
   b. Trimetazidine
   c. Nicorandil
   d. Ramipril

Q4. Which of the following does not reduce mortality in hypertension with angina pectoris?
   a. Atorvastatin
   b. Isosorbide mononitrate
   c. Ramipril
   d. Aspirin

Q5. Which of the following statement is incorrect?
   a. Angiotensin-converting enzyme (ACE) inhibitors have significant antianginal properties
   b. Beta-blockers can safely be combined with amlodipine
   c. Oral nitrates do not have antihypertensive effects
   d. Diuretics are usually a low-order choice in patients with hypertension and angina pectoris

Ans. 1-b, 2-d, 3-b, 4-b, 5-a

DISCUSSION

Hypertension is a major independent and modifiable risk factor for coronary artery disease (CAD). As per the findings of INTERHEART study, hypertension was accountable for 17.9% of the population attributable risk of several cardiovascular (CV) risk factors for CAD.

Coronary artery disease and systemic hypertension are age-dependent risk factors for adverse events. The major predictor of ischemic heart disease (IHD) risk before the age of 50 years is diastolic blood pressure (DBP). While in individuals >60 years, systolic blood pressure (SBP) is more significant. Among the individuals who are of age 60 years or more, there exists an inverse relationship between DBP and CAD risk, and pulse pressure becomes the strongest predictor for CAD. For each 20 mm Hg increase in SBP (or for each 10 mm Hg rise in DBP), the risk of a fatal coronary event doubles.

In patients with hypertension, reduction of BP results in rapid decrease in CV risk. A 10 mm Hg lower usual SBP (or a 5 mm Hg lower usual DBP) is related to a 40–50% reduced risk of death caused due to CAD.

Pathogenesis of Coronary Artery Disease: The Importance of Hypertension

Multiple systemic effects are caused by hypertension that results in end-organ damage. It has been shown to cause reduced vascular compliance as well as endothelial injury. In the pathogenesis of atherosclerosis as well as CAD, endothelial injury has been shown to be one of the major mechanisms.

The renin–angiotensin–aldosterone system (RAAS) is another significant mechanism of hypertension causing CAD. Angiotensin II elevates BP and the reactive oxygen species generation, which tend to oppose the beneficial vascular effects of nitric oxide. It has been shown that angiotensin II enhances the arterial wall stiffness, and therefore results in impairment of vascular compliance. Angiotensin II also helps in the development of insulin resistance and stimulates the production of proinflammatory molecules that result in vascular inflammation as well as coagulopathy.

There is an association of hypertension with enhanced sympathetic activity that results in increase in levels of plasma norepinephrine and raised BP, cardiac output, heart rate (HR), and reabsorption of renal tubular sodium. Such changes lead to a vicious cycle, along with a consequent rise in RAAS activity further resulting in hypertension as well as CAD.

Evaluation

Assess the likelihood of clinically significant CAD on the basis of the following factors: The character of the chest pain (typical, atypical, or nonanginal), age, sex, other risk factors, Q wave or ST-T wave changes on ECG, and baseline echocardiogram.

Treatment

It has been reported by meta-analyses of antihypertensive trials that reduction of BP is more essential than the specific drug class that is used for the primary prevention of the complications of hypertension, including CAD. For achieving and sustaining effective long-term control of BP, the typical requirement is of a combination antihypertensive drug therapy. For the primary prevention of CAD, there exists no evidence that supports initiation of treatment with any one antihypertensive drug class over another. On the contrary, not all drug classes have been proven to confer same level of benefit for secondary protection.

Among patients having chronic CAD, the management of hypertension is aimed to decrease the frequency as well as duration of myocardial ischemia; prevent myocardial infarction (MI), stroke, and death; and the amelioration of symptoms.

Changing lifestyle and adopting a heart healthy approach are important. Attention needs to be paid to the diet, intake of sodium, cessation of smoking, moderate intake of alcohol, weight reduction, regular exercise, good glycemic control, antiplatelet therapy, and lipid management. Pharmacological management is essentially needed.

A reasonable BP target for hypertensive patients with demonstrated CAD is <140/90 mm Hg.

Beta-blockers

These are the first choice of drugs for the treatment of hypertension among patients who have CAD that causes angina. They alleviate ischemia and angina primarily as a function of their negative inotropic and chronotropic actions. The reduced HR enhances the diastolic filling time for coronary perfusion. Beta-blockers also inhibit release of renin from juxtaglomerular apparatus. The beta-blockers that are used most frequently include cardioselective ($\beta 1$) agents without intrinsic sympathomimetic activity.

According to the recent ACC Foundation/AHA guidelines, beta-blocker therapy is recommended for patients having normal LV function after acute coronary syndrome (ACS) (Class I) or MI, particularly bisoprolol, carvedilol, or metoprolol in all patients who have LV systolic dysfunction [ejection fraction (EF) ≤40%)] or who have previous MI or HF if not contraindicated (Class I). It is also recommended to start beta-blockers and continue them for 3 years among all the patients who have normal LV function following ACS or MI.

Calcium Channel Blockers

Calcium channel blockers (CCBs), as a class, cause reduction in the myocardial oxygen demand by reducing the peripheral vascular resistance and BP and increasing myocardial oxygen supply by coronary vasodilation. The nondihydropyridine agents (e.g., verapamil, diltiazem) also reduce the sinus node discharge rate as well as slow atrioventricular nodal conduction.

For providing relief of symptoms, CCBs should be prescribed when beta-blockers are contraindicated or in cases where beta-blockers lead to unacceptable side effects in patients with stable angina (Class IIa). In the conditions when BP remains elevated, angina persists, or when drug side effects or contraindications mandate, CCBs are added to, or substituted for, beta-blockers.

For preventing excessive bradycardia, the long-acting dihydropyridine agents are preferred over nondihydropyridines (such as verapamil or diltiazem) for use along with beta-blockers. Among patients who have HF or LV systolic dysfunction, the use of diltiazem or verapamil should be avoided, and short-acting nifedipine should not be used as it leads to reflex sympathetic activation as well as worsening of myocardial ischemia. They do not prevent cardiovascular events among patients who have established CAD.

Angiotensin-converting Enzyme Inhibitors

The two clinical trials which support the use of ACE inhibitors for the management of patients who have stable CAD are—HOPE (Heart Outcomes Prevention Evaluation) study and EUROPA (European Trial on Reduction of Cardiac events with Perindopril in Stable Coronary Artery Disease). The HOPE study included high-risk individuals, out of which 80% had CAD and a reduction in CVD end points by 20–25%. In the EUROPA study, there was a 20% relative risk reduction among patients who have established CAD.

It is recommended to prescribe ACE inhibitors in all the CAD patients who have stable angina and also diabetes mellitus (DM), hypertension (HTN), an LVEF ≤40%, or chronic kidney disease (CKD) unless contraindicated (Class I).

Angiotensin II Receptor Blockers
It is recommended to prescribe ARBs in all the patients who have stable angina with DM, HTN, CKD, or reduced ejection fraction have indications for, but are intolerant to, ACE inhibitors (Class I). In patients with STEMI who are intolerant of ACE inhibitors and have HF or an EF <0.40 (Class I), ARBs are recommended at the time of hospitalization as well as at discharge. It is not recommended to use the combination of ARBs and ACE inhibitors.

Diuretics
As reported in the MRC (Medical Research Council) trial, the Veterans Administration studies, and ALLHAT (Antihypertensive and Lipid Lowering Treatment to Prevent Heart Attack Trial) and SHEP (Systolic Hypertension in the Elderly Program) SHEP and ALLHAT trials, thiazide diuretics and thiazide-like diuretics decrease cardiovascular events. But, because of the metabolic side effects related to thiazides, they are still used with caution in individuals with CAD.

Nitrates
Long-acting nitrates are recommended for the relief from symptoms in case beta-blockers are ineffective or contraindicated or result in undesirable side effects among patients who have stable angina (Class I). Nitrates should not be prescribed in combination with phosphodiesterase inhibitors (such as sildenafil). Nitrates have generally not been shown to be of use in the management of hypertension.

■ KEY POINTS
- The aim of the management of symptomatic CAD is at providing the relief of the angina as well as preventing both the progression of CAD and coronary events.
- Beta-blockers, CCBs, and nitrates are the mainstays of treatment of angina. In such patients, to prevent cardiovascular events, pharmacological strategies include antiplatelet drugs, ACE inhibitors, ARBs, beta-blockers (specifically after MI), CCBs, thiazide and thiazide-like diuretics, and drugs for the treatment of dyslipidemia.
- According to the recommendation of the recent ACC/AHA (American College of Cardiology/American Heart Association) guidelines, ACE inhibitors and/or beta-blockers, along with drugs like CCBs or thiazide diuretics, should be prescribed for the management of high BP among patients who have stable IHD.

■ SUGGESTED READING
1. Rosendorff C, Lackland DT, Allison M, et al. Treatment of hypertension in patients with coronary artery disease: A scientific statement from the American Heart Association, American College of Cardiology, and American Society of Hypertension. J Am Coll Cardiol. 2015;65(18).

> **CASE 3: Hypertension and Heart Failure**
>
> A 60-year-old hypertensive man was admitted to the hospital with worsening dyspnea from New York Heart Association (NYHA) Class II to NYHA Class III over past 3 months, and increased to NYHA Class IV since morning. He had been on tablet amlodipine 5 mg since past 5 years with no regular visits to physician.
>
> On examination, the heart rate was 108 beats/min, blood pressure was 160/94 mm Hg, and respiratory rate was 28 breaths/min. Respiratory system revealed bilateral rales covering half of lung fields. On cardiovascular examination, S_3 was present.
>
> An electrocardiogram (ECG) revealed poor progression of R-waves in precordial leads, with transition zone in V_5.
>
> Chest X-ray showed cardiomegaly with signs of pulmonary venous hypertension (PVH).
>
> Baseline echocardiography showed dilated left ventricle (LV) cavity (60 mm) with global hypokinesia of left ventricle with LV ejection fraction (LVEF) = 36%. Her resting pulmonary artery systolic pressure (PASP) was 50 mm Hg.

Q1. Which of the following statements is true?
   a. Raised levels of atrial natriuretic peptide (ANP) are thought to be beneficial in heart failure
   b. A third heart sound is an uncommon finding
   c. Heart looks small on plain posteroanterior chest radiograph
   d. All diuretics used in treatment of heart failure potentially cause hypokalemia

Q2. First-line agent used in treating congestive heart failure:
   a. Hydralazine
   b. Dobutamine
   c. Angiotensin-converting enzyme (ACE) inhibitors
   d. Calcium channel blockers (CCBs)

Q3. Management of this patient should include all except:
   a. Add ACE inhibitor or angiotensin II receptor blocker (ARB) to control blood pressure
   b. Restriction of salt and activity
   c. Combination of loop diuretic and aldosterone antagonist
   d. Increase the dose of amlodipine

Q4. Effect of sacubitril/valsartan on natriuretic peptides is:
   a. Decrease in B-type natriuretic peptide (BNP) and pro-B-type natriuretic peptide (NT-proBNP)
   b. Increase in BNP and NT-proBNP
   c. Increase in BNP and decrease in NT-proBNP
   d. Decrease in BNP and increase in NT-proBNP

Q5. Which of the following statements is wrong about digoxin in heart failure?
   a. No mortality benefit
   b. Reduces symptoms
   c. Reduces recurrent hospitalizations
   d. Class I recommendation

Ans. 1-a, 2-c, 3-d, 4-c, 5-d

DISCUSSION

Hypertension is the most prevalent modifiable risk factor for the development of heart failure (HF), both because hypertension increases cardiac work, which leads to the development of left ventricular hypertrophy (LVH) (**Fig. 1**).

In hypertensive patients, there is variation in incidence of HF as per the population as well as follow-up duration. For example, in the ACCOMPLISH trial, nearly 2% of the high-risk hypertensive patients developed HF at 3 years. In the ALLHAT study, during an average follow-up of 9 years, nearly 5.4% individuals developed HF in the high-risk hypertensive population.

Unlike the pattern observed in the general population, where there is poor prognosis in individuals with hypertension as compared to the normotensive individuals, an elevated BP before treatment is a predictor of better survival among patients having HF. This correlation is possibly a result of the fact that more severe cardiac dysfunction results in a decrease in systemic BP, thus rendering low BP to be a marker for more advanced HF.

Treatment of hypertension in patients with HF must take into account the type of HF that is present. In systolic dysfunction, the primary abnormality is the impairment of cardiac contractility. In diastolic dysfunction, there is a limitation to diastolic filling and thus in forward output due to increased ventricular stiffness.

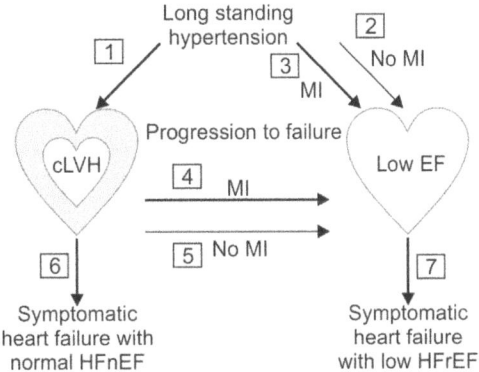

(cLVH: concentric LVH; EF: ejection fraction; MI: myocardial infarction)

Fig. 1: Pathways in the progression from hypertension to heart failure.

Treatment of Hypertension in Patients with HFrEF (Flowchart 1, Table 1)

The goals of antihypertensive therapy in the setting of reduced EF are to reduce both preload (to diminish congestive symptoms) using diuretics and after load (to improve cardiac output) using vasodilators [renin–angiotensin–aldosterone system (RAAS)]. Neurohormonal blockade, with beta-blockers or antagonists of the RAAS, also improves cardiac contractility and lower blood pressure.

These patients should be treated, if possible, with an angiotensin-converting enzyme (ACE) inhibitor [or, alternatively, an ARB or angiotensin receptor neprilysin inhibitor (ARNI)], a beta-blocker, and a mineralocorticoid receptor

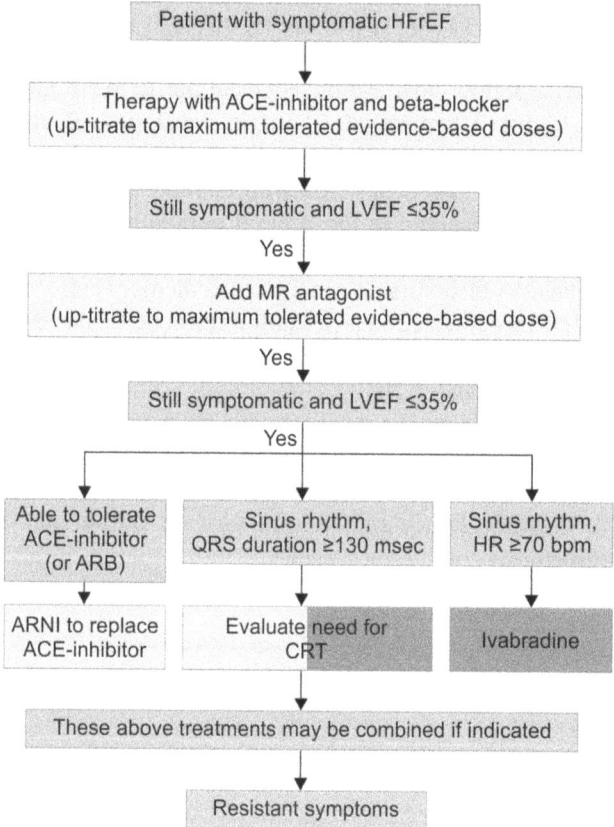

(ACE: angiotensin-converting enzyme; ARB: angiotensin II receptor blocker; ARNI: angiotensin-receptor neprilysin inhibitor; CRT: cardiac resynchronization therapy; LVEF: left ventricular ejection fraction; HR: heart rate)

Flowchart 1: Algorithm for a patient with symptomatic heart failure with reduced ejection fraction (HFrEF).

TABLE 1: Evidence-based doses of disease-modifying drugs HFrEF.

	Starting dose (mg)	Target dose (mg)		Starting dose (mg)	Target dose (mg)
ACE inhibitor			**ARBs**		
Enalapril	2.5 bid	10–20 bid	Candesartan	4–8 od	32 od
Lisinopril	2.5–5.0 od	20–35 od	Valsartan	40 bid	160 bid
Ramipril	2.5 od	10 od	Losartan	50 od	150 od
Beta-blockers			**MRAs**		
Bisoprolol	1.25 od	10 od	Eplerenone	25 od	50 od
Carvedilol	3.125 bid	25 bid	Spironolactone	25 od	50 od
Metoprolol succinate (CR/XL)	12.5–25 od	200 od	**ARNI**		
Nebivolol	1.25 od	10 od	Sacubitril/ Valsartan	49/51 bid	97/103 bid

(ACE: angiotensin-converting enzyme; ARB: angiotensin receptor blocker; ARNI: angiotensin-receptor neprilysin inhibitor; MRA: mineralocorticoid receptor antagonist)

antagonist. In addition to the mortality benefit associated with this regimen in patients with HFrEF, many patients will experience a minor to moderate improvement in their EF, with occasional patients experiencing substantial improvement.

Diuretics are used to treat symptomatic hypervolemia (pulmonary and/or peripheral edema) or to further reduce blood pressure, if needed, in hypervolemic patients.

Angiotensin-converting enzyme inhibitors, when given to the patients with mild to advanced heart failure, result in enhanced cardiac output, reduced congestive symptoms, decreased rate of progressive cardiac dysfunction as well as reduced cardiovascular mortality. ACE inhibitors also help patients who have asymptomatic left ventricular dysfunction. In spite of these beneficial cardiovascular effects, ACE inhibitors usually do not improve renal function in patients with HF. In contrast, an increase in the plasma creatinine concentration takes place in nearly 30% cases. This complication is most likely to take place in those patients in whom maintaining the glomerular filtration rate is dependent on angiotensin II, e.g., individuals taking high-dose diuretic therapy. Such patients also have an increased risk of first-dose hypotension. The ACE inhibitor does not generally need to be discontinued unless there is a large increase in plasma creatinine or the plasma creatinine continues to rise.

Angiotensin II receptor blocking drugs are most often used in patients who are intolerant of ACE inhibitors or are already taking an ARB for some other reason. An ARB should not be combined with an ACE inhibitor.

In patients who have symptomatic HF and reduced EF, drugs that combine an ARB with a neprilysin inhibitor may be used in place of an ACE inhibitor or ARB.

It has been shown that in patients with mild to advanced HF, some of the beta-blockers, such as bisoprolol, carvedilol, and metoprolol, improve overall and event-free survival. The improvement in survival is additive to that induced by ACE inhibitors. Among the patients who have New York Heart Association (NYHA) class II–IV HF and have been stabilized on an ACE inhibitor as well as diuretics, beta-blocker therapy should be taken into consideration, independent of hypertension. In the patients who have HF, carvedilol may be specifically beneficial for reducing blood pressure.

In addition to fluid removal with loop diuretics, mineralocorticoid receptor antagonists [spironolactone (25 mg) or eplerenone at a dose of 50 mg/day] have been shown to improve survival in patients with advanced HF. There is evidence for at least two mechanisms of benefit: An elevation in the serum potassium concentration, and prevention of the toxic effect of hyperaldosteronism on the heart.

Diuretic therapy for signs of fluid overload (pulmonary and/or peripheral edema) is usually initiated with a loop diuretic (e.g., furosemide). The fall in intracardiac filling pressure that results from diuretic-induced fluid removal may lower blood pressure, particularly when the renin–angiotensin system is inhibited. In hypervolemic individuals, cardiac output is usually not affected, although excessive diuresis may reduce cardiac output.

Hydralazine/nitrates: The combination of hydralazine and isosorbide dinitrate is found to be particularly effective in blacks with HF who were already being treated with standard therapies. However, it requires multiple daily doses and may produce more side effects than an ACE inhibitor.

Calcium channel blockers (CCBs): Studies show a deleterious decrease in cardiac function of many CCBs in patients with HF. Amlodipine and felodipine, however, do not decrease cardiac function or increase mortality. Thus, while there is no direct role for these drugs in the management of HF, amlodipine and felodipine appear to be safe and well tolerated and can be used for the treatment of coexisting hypertension.

KEY POINTS

- In case blood pressure is not controlled with an ACE inhibitor (or an ARB), the additional BP lowering agents considered to be safe in systolic HF include a beta-blocker, a mineralocorticoid receptor antagonist and a diuretic, and then hydralazine and amlodipine (or felodipine).

> **CASE 4: Hypertension and Acute Myocardial Infarction**
>
> A 52-year-old diabetic man presented with sudden onset chest pain to the emergency. The pain started 2 hours back. Pain was retrosternal in location, radiating to both shoulders, and was associated with vomiting.
>
> On examination, the heart rate was 94 beats/min, blood pressure was 200/110 mm Hg, and respiratory rate was 18 breaths/min.
>
> The electrocardiogram demonstrated ST elevation in V_1–V_4 with tall T waves.
>
> Bedside echocardiography showed akinesia of basal mid and apical part of the septum with LV ejection fraction (LVEF) of 45%. No mitral regurgitation (MR) was present and no other mechanical complication was seen.

Q1. Which of the following statement is TRUE regarding management of this patient?
   a. BP should be immediately lowered to 120/80 mm Hg, irrespective of reperfusion strategy
   b. Significant hypertension at initial evaluation in an absolute contraindication for thrombolysis
   c. Primary percutaneous coronary intervention (PCI) can be safely performed
   d. Antiplatelets have to be administered only when BP is controlled

Q2. Which of the following factor(s) is associated with increased risk of rupture of the interventricular septum? [Post myocardial infarction (MI) ventricular septal defects (VSD)]
   a. Advanced age
   b. Hypertension
   c. Anterior location of infarction
   d. All of the above

Q3. Left ventricular hypertrophy in patients presenting with myocardial infarction (MI) predicts:
   a. Favorable outcome
   b. Increased risk of sudden death
   c. Less ventricular remodeling
   d. Lesser adverse events

Q4. Which of the following statements is not true for the management of this patient?
   a. IV nitroglycerin with oral antihypertensive agents will be a good choice
   b. Sodium nitroprusside infusion will be the best choice
   c. IV beta-blockers (metoprolol) can be used especially if marked tachycardia is present
   d. Angiotensin-converting enzyme (ACE) inhibitors should be started from day one in such a patient

Q5. Risk reduction is seen with all of the following anti-hypertensive agents when used in acute myocardial infarction, except:
   a. Beta-blockers
   b. Diuretics
   c. ACE inhibitors
   d. ARBs

Ans. 1-c, 2-d, 3-b, 4-b, 5-b

DISCUSSION

The prevalence of antecedent hypertension among patients having acute myocardial infarction (AMI) is in the range of 31–59%. There is an increase in prevalence of hypertension along with increasing age in patients with acute coronary syndrome (ACS); prevalence rates of hypertension approximately double in the individuals >75 years of age as compared to those <45 years of age. There is an association of antecedent hypertension with higher rates of death as well as morbid events in the early- and long-term course of AMI.

On contrary to ominous implications carried by antecedent hypertension, BP values in hypertensive range at onset of AMI carry favorable long-term prognosis. In trials, it was observed that an inverse relationship between mortality and systolic blood pressure at admission was maintained even after excluding participants who died in the course of hospitalization and those who already had or did develop a diagnosis of chronic heart failure (CHF) and after accounting for the increased risk of hemorrhagic stroke of thrombolytic treatment in presence of increased systolic blood pressure.

According to the findings of GUSTO IIb and PURSUIT trials, there was a strong association of a very low systolic blood pressure (90 mm Hg or less) with 48-hour and 30-day mortality; however, little difference was noted in mortality between patients with an elevated systolic blood pressure (>140 mm Hg) and patients who have a normal or prehypertensive range of systolic blood pressure (121–140 mm Hg).

Although uncontrolled hypertension does not appear to significantly increase in-hospital mortality in patients with AMI, it is a major risk factor for intracranial hemorrhage. BP should be reduced to <160/110 mm Hg before administration of thrombolysis, as significant hypertension is a relative contraindication for it. If available, primary angioplasty is an option for reperfusion in patients with high BP.

There is a U-shaped association between blood pressure and in-hospital bleeding; there is excess bleeding for both the patients who have hypertension and those who have hypotension. As per findings of CRUSADE registry, bleeding rates were lowest in patients with admission systolic blood pressure between 120 and 180 mm Hg and increased progressively with pressures above and below these ranges.

Though, all of the data is observational and has several limitations, the consistent associations found between hypotension and both mortality and bleeding suggest that avoidance of hypotension should be an important treatment principle in ACS patients.

Among patients with AMI, left ventricular hypertrophy (LVH) that was evaluated either by ECG or by echographic criteria predicted an enhanced risk of sudden death as well as left ventricular remodeling in the early phase and the long-term recovery. In the presence of concentric LVH, adverse events occurred more frequently as compared to the normal geometry. Other proischemic mechanisms of LVH are reduction in coronary reserve due to vascular remodeling of coronary resistance-sized arterioles, impairment in endothelial-mediated vasorelaxation, and disturbance in ischemic preconditioning.

General Principles of Blood Pressure Management in the Patient with Acute Myocardial Infarction

Treatment should be aimed at relieving symptoms, protecting the ischemic but potentially viable myocardial tissue and reducing mortality. Alteration of the balance between the myocardial oxygen supply and the demand is the cornerstone of the management. Increase in BP results in increased myocardial oxygen demand; however, rapid and excessive decrease of the diastolic blood pressure leads to impaired coronary blood flow as well as oxygen supply. Additionally, in these patients, there is vasomotor instability along with an enhanced tendency to exaggerating response to antihypertensive therapy.

There is limited specific data of BP lowering among patients who have AMI. The focus of the selection of antihypertensive agents is based on selection of drugs having a proven evidence base for risk reduction for patients having ACS independently of lowering of BP. These drugs include ACE inhibitors [or angiotensin receptor blockers (ARBs)], beta-blockers, and, in particular patients, aldosterone antagonists; there should be typical titration of these drugs to full doses before other agents.

There are no established therapeutic targets for BP particularly for patients having ACS. According to current guidelines, target of BP should be <140/90 mm Hg; however, this is applicable more to secondary prevention as compared to the hypertension management in the acute phase of myocardial infarction. There may be fluctuation in BP early after myocardial infarction. Therefore, control of pain and clinical stabilization is particularly targeted. Lowering of BP should be done slowly; it is advised to have caution for avoiding reductions in diastolic blood pressure to <60 mm Hg as this may decrease coronary perfusion as well as worsen ischemia.

Specific Antihypertensive Agents in Acute Coronary Syndrome

Nitroglycerin

For decades, nitroglycerin has been a cornerstone of treatment. In the patient with hypertension having AMI, nitroglycerin is considered to be effective in providing relief of symptoms of ischemia as well as pulmonary congestion; it is moderately effective in reducing arterial BP. However, evidence from clinical trial does not favor an impact of nitrates on the outcomes in AMI. Therefore, it is not recommended by ACC/AHA (American College of Cardiology/American Heart Association) guidelines for ST-segment elevation myocardial infarction (STEMI) to use nitroglycerin for reducing events, and it should only be used for relieving ischemic pain or acute hypertension or for managing pulmonary congestion. Among patients who have inferior STEMI, nitrates should be used cautiously. These agents are contraindicated in cases when right ventricular infarction is present. It is suggested not to use nitroglycerin at the expense of agents with established advantages on outcomes (e.g., beta-blockers or ACE inhibitors).

Beta-blockers

There is an ability of beta-blockers to decrease heart rate as well as BP and therefore myocardial oxygen demand. Beta-blockers were amongst the first therapies that are shown to decrease infarct size. Through antiarrhythmic effects and prevention of myocardial rupture, beta-blockers decrease early sudden death post MI. In several trials, the advantages of long-term post discharge beta-blockers have been shown among patients who have STEMI. So, in patients having ACS, use of beta-blockers is presently considered to be a quality performance measure. Beta-blockers should be started early and continued for minimum 3 years following AMI. IV beta-blockers are used only in young patients with anterior infarcts and marked sinus tachycardia and hypertension especially amongst those who are in Killip's class I.

According to the recommendations by current ACC/AHA guidelines, once it is proved that the patient is in stable condition and there exists no contraindications, oral beta-blockade should be initiated within the first 24 hours. Short-acting cardioselective (β1-selective) beta-blockers without intrinsic sympathomimetic activity (e.g., bisoprolol or metoprolol) are preferred. Carvedilol (that also blocks α1 and β2 adrenergic receptors) possesses more potent BP-reducing effects, and so, it is a good option for patients who have AMI as well as severe hypertension.

Calcium Channel Blockers

In the setting of acute STEMI, calcium channel blockers (CCBs) generally are not found to be beneficial. Rapid-release form of nifedipine showed an increased mortality among patients who were treated with this agent after MI. The non dihydropyridine agents, diltiazem and verapamil, are also not recommended in acute STEMI. According to recommendation by AHA/ACC guidelines, among patients who have continuing or frequently recurring ischemia when beta-blockers are contraindicated, an alternative that may be used is a non-dihydropyridine CCB (diltiazem or verapamil) when there is absence of significant LV dysfunction or other contraindications.

Evidence for the utility of dihydropyridine CCBs is limited with potential to cause hypotension. These agents may effectively lower BP and relieve ischemic symptoms.

Angiotensin-converting Enzyme Inhibitors and Angiotensin Receptor Blockers

Angiotensin-converting enzyme inhibitors, indicated for most patients, are considered to be a preferable option for management of BP. They result in reduction of infarct expansion, prevention of LV remodeling as well as chamber dilatation, which helps in preventing downstream sequelae (e.g., heart failure, ventricular arrhythmia, or even myocardial rupture). As reported in the GISSI-3, and ISIS-4 trials, a benefit was observed by early administration of ACE inhibitors, with absolute reductions in mortality of 0.5%, 0.8%, and 0.5%, respectively noted as early as 4 weeks following AMI.

If ACE inhibitors are initiated later after MI in patients who have LV dysfunction and are continued for a longer term, their advantages are even more robust. As reported in long-term trials, there was reduction in mortality rates by nearly 20%.

Angiotensin receptor blockers are a useful alternative to ACE inhibitors in patients with an ACE inhibitor contraindication or intolerance. These are a first-line alternatives for ACE inhibitor-intolerant patients.

Aldosterone Antagonists

Aldosterone is not completely suppressed even in patients who are receiving high doses of ACE inhibitors. Aldosterone is believed contribute to both adverse ventricular remodeling as well as myocardial fibrosis following an MI. It has been shown that the aldosterone antagonists decrease cardiovascular and overall mortality, along with decreasing sudden cardiac death also.

It is recommended to avoid aldosterone antagonists among patients who have significantly increased levels of serum creatinine (men: ≥ 2.5 mg/dL; women: ≥ 2.0 mg/dL) or increased levels of potassium (≥ 5.0 mEq/L), as using these agents poses a serious risk of hyperkalemia among those patients who have an estimated creatinine clearance of <50 mL/min. It is necessary to perform close clinical and laboratory follow-up in the patients who receive treatment with aldosterone antagonists for long term.

Mineralocorticoid antagonists are underused among evidence-based medications after MI. This probably shows appropriate concerns related to the risk for hyperkalemia associated with such agents. With careful follow-up, these highly effective as well as economical agents can be received by the patients safely.

Diuretics

There is a main role of thiazide and thiazide-type diuretics in the long-term control of BP; however, in patients with ACS, diuretics are used mainly for patients who have evidence of enhanced pulmonary venous congestion, filling pressures, or heart failure. Regarding hypokalemia, specific attention is required, as it can precipitate arrhythmias following ACS. As compared to thiazide and thiazide-type diuretics, loop diuretics are preferred in patients who have ACS with heart failure (NYHA class III or IV) or among patients having CKD and an estimated glomerular filtration rate of <45 mL/min.

KEY POINTS

- There is high prevalence of hypertension in patients who have ACS, specifically with advancement of age.
- Most of the patients will respond to standard methods of controlling hypertension. It is recommended to select particular agents having an established evidence base for reduction of risk in ACS. Such agents are ACE inhibitors, beta-blockers, or ARBs, and, in some of the selected patients—aldosterone antagonists.
- Nitrates do not affect the natural history of ACS. In patients with hypertension and ACS, nitrates are beneficial, specifically when ongoing ischemia or pulmonary congestion is present. Particular care should be taken to avoid hypotension, with the risk of worsening myocardial ischemia. The advantages of treating hypertension in the ACS setting are reasonable; however, the main impact on long-term morbidity as well as mortality is dependent on the efficacy of continuous outpatient control of BP after the initiation of effective therapy in the hospital.

CASE 5: Hypertension and Atrial Fibrillation

A 58-year-old female, known diabetic and hypertensive, presented with complaints of vertigo and multiple episodes of vomiting, associated with headache.

On examination, her heart rate was 126 beats/min, irregularly irregular, blood pressure (BP) was 160/100 mm Hg, and respiratory rate was 18 breaths/min.

On central nervous system examination, 5-hydroxymethylfurfural (HMF) was normal. Cerebellar signs on right side were found to be positive. Power was 5/5 in both upper and lower limbs. Respiratory system and cardiovascular examinations were normal.

An electrocardiogram demonstrated atrial fibrillation (AF):
- Two-dimensional magnetic resonance imaging (2D MRI) brain revealed multiple infarcts in posterior circulation territory.
- 2D echocardiography showed normal left ventricular (LV) function with left atrial (LA) moderately dilated. No LA/LA appendage (LAA) could be visualized on transthoracic echocardiography.

Q1. The management of this patient should include all except:
  a. Long-term anticoagulation with vitamin K antagonist to maintain INR between 2 and 3
  b. Good blood pressure control to <140/90 mm Hg
  c. Immediate cardioversion to revert the arrhythmia to sinus rhythm
  d. Stroke rehabilitation and regular physiotherapy

Q2. As per CHA2DS$_2$-VaSc score, what is annual risk of recurrent stroke in this patient?
   a. <1%
   b. 1–5%
   c. 5–10%
   d. >10%

Q3. CHA2DS$_2$-VaSc score includes all except:
   a. Coronary artery disease
   b. Hypertension
   c. Age
   d. Diabetes

Q4. This patient had atrial fibrillation and a stroke. What is the recommended anticoagulant therapy?
   a. Aspirin 75 mg/day
   b. Aspirin 75 mg/day plus clopidogrel 75 mg/day
   c. Vitamin K antagonist
   d. Vitamin K antagonist plus aspirin 75 mg/day

Q5. Which of the following is true regarding the use of antihypertensive agents in atrial fibrillation?
   a. Blood pressure is the main goal
   b. Drugs blocking the renin–angiotensin–aldosterone system (RAAS) reduce the risk of new-onset atrial fibrillation
   c. Beta-blockers are effective for rate control
   d. All of the above

Ans. 1-c, 2-c, 3-a, 4-c, 5-d

DISCUSSION

Atrial fibrillation (AF) is considered to be the most common clinically significant sustained cardiac arrhythmia that takes place among 1–2% of the general population. In India, there is not much epidemiology data on AF, apart from some knowledge from the REALIZE and RELY studies (Indian cohort).

Hypertension as such enhances the risk of AF by nearly 2-fold. As compared to other risk factors, hypertension is accountable for more cases of AF; this was observed in 50–80% of patients in several AF trials.

It has been shown that hypertension generally coexists along with several conditions associated with AF, 82% of chronic kidney disease patients, 77% of patients with diabetes, 73% of coronary artery disease patients, 72% of stroke patients, 71% of patients with heart failure, and 62% patients with metabolic syndrome. As reported by recent studies, the progression of renal dysfunction is a strong predictor of new-onset atrial fibrillation in patients with hypertension, independently of left ventricular hypertrophy (LVH) and left atrial dilatation.

Long-standing hypertension, particularly when suboptimally controlled, results in LVH, structural changes and the left atrium enlargement, heterogeneity of atrial conduction as well as fibrosis, all of which can result in the development of AF.

In all the stages of the cardiovascular disease (CVD) continuum, AF may take place. Presence of several risk factors in the early stages (such as diabetes, obesity, and hypertension) may predispose patients to AF; however, the development of subclinical as well as clinical organ damage not only predisposes patients to AF, but also the presence of AF may in turn increase the risk of CVD.

Atrial fibrillation is the most common arrhythmia in patients with heart failure and it worsens prognosis. Not only the presence of atrial fibrillation but also the new onset of atrial fibrillation carries a higher risk in patients with heart failure. In the patients having new-onset AF, the rate of in-hospital mortality is significantly high. Atrial fibrillation is considered to be the major cause of hospitalizations for arrhythmias and it is accountable for nearly one-third of the cases of hospitalizations for heart rhythm disturbances.

Among patients who have AF along with history of hypertension, the increase in the annual incidence of stroke is threefold in comparison with individuals without a history of hypertension. Arrhythmia can be asymptomatic in nearly 33% of the patients with AF. According to the Holter monitoring studies, as compared to the symptomatic episodes, the asymptomatic episodes of paroxysmal AF are 10–12 times more common.

An independent risk factor for death is AF. Individuals having AF have a 40–90% more risk of overall mortality in comparison with those with normal sinus rhythm. It is usually associated with significant CV disorders, such as heart failure and stroke. AF is accountable for nearly 15–20% of all ischemic strokes; it enhances the risk of stroke 4- to 5-fold; it is an independent risk factor for severity and recurrence of ischemic stroke. Worsening of the cognitive function, enhanced risk of hospitalization as well as cost, and impairment in quality of life are the other outcomes of AF.

Diagnostic Approach

Symptoms caused by AF include dizziness, palpitations, anxiety, mild shortness of breath, and generalized weakness. However, nearly 90% AF episodes can be asymptomatic. More serious signs and symptoms (e.g., severe shortness of breath, hemodynamic instability, and chest pain) can be because of associated cardiac diseases like heart failure or ischemic heart disease. The recommended first step is 12-lead electrocardiogram (ECG). An echocardiogram should be considered for hypertensive patients. Several cardiac diseases (such as heart failure, ischemic heart disease, and valvular diseases) are associated with AF. So, evaluation of levels of B-type natriuretic peptide and serum cardiac biomarkers should be considered after the confirmation of diagnosis of AF.

Atrial fibrillation is classified as following:
- *First diagnosed*: Regardless of the duration
- *Paroxysmal*: Self-terminating generally within 48 hours or within <7 days
- *Persistent*: Lasts >7 days or need termination by cardioversion
- *Permanent*: Remains for >1 year

A silent AF can be detected from an AF-associated complication as first manifestation or it can be diagnosed by an opportunistic ECG.

Risk Stratification and Thromboembolism

Atrial fibrillation is found to be associated with an enhanced risk of thromboembolism leading to stroke, peripheral embolization, or transient ischemic attack. The predictive rule that is used most commonly is $CHADS_2$ (that stands for Congestive heart failure, Hypertension, Age, Diabetes, Stroke) score. In the $CHADS_2$ index, 1 point is assigned each for a history of heart failure, hypertension, age >75 years and diabetes, and 2 points are assigned for a history of transient ischemic attack or stroke.

Several independent cohorts have validated a refined version of the original $CHADS_2$ score, which is known as $CHA2DS_2$-VASc score. The $CHADS_2$ score is surpassed by the $CHA2DS_2$-VASc score in identification of "truly low-risk" patients in whom antithrombotic therapy is not required, while individuals having minimum one risk factor for stroke should be considered for oral anticoagulation. **Figure 1** shows annual risk of stroke.

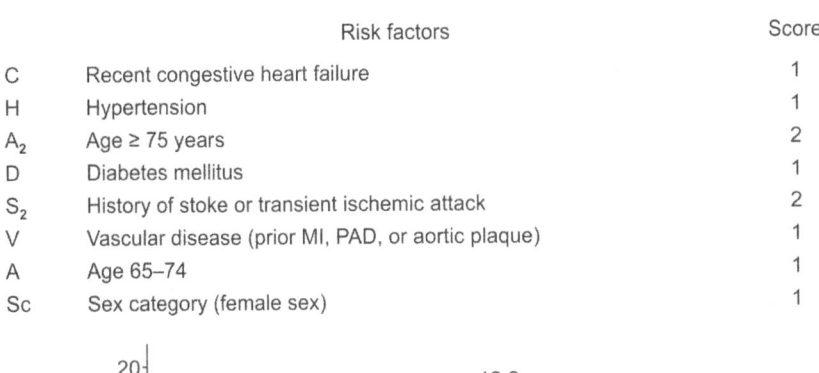

	Risk factors	Score
C	Recent congestive heart failure	1
H	Hypertension	1
A_2	Age ≥ 75 years	2
D	Diabetes mellitus	1
S_2	History of stoke or transient ischemic attack	2
V	Vascular disease (prior MI, PAD, or aortic plaque)	1
A	Age 65–74	1
Sc	Sex category (female sex)	1

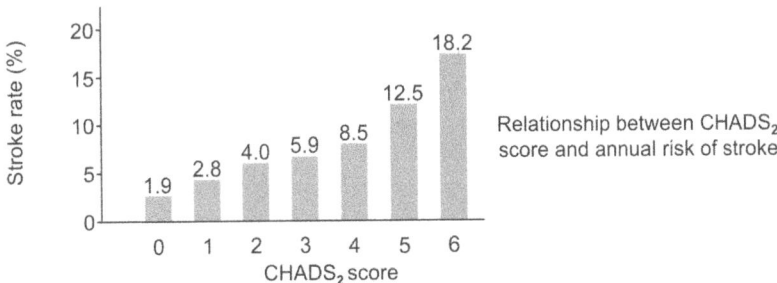

Relationship between $CHADS_2$ score and annual risk of stroke

(MI: myocardial infarction; PAD: peripheral artery disease)

Fig. 1: $CHA2DS_2$-VASc score and annual risk of stroke.

Management

Management of the patients who have AF is directed at prevention of AF by regulating the risk factors associated with the development of AF, decreasing the symptoms, and at avoiding severe complications that are related to AF.

Atrial Fibrillation and Antihypertensive Treatment

Risk for AF is decreased by the antihypertensive drugs primarily by reducing elevated BP. There exist few prospective studies related to the development of AF in patients with hypertension; however, many secondary analyses of large randomized trials as well as few meta-analyses exist.

The primary aim in patients having hypertension and atrial fibrillation is reduction of BP per se. Drugs that block the RAAS decrease the risk of new-onset AF. However, this effect has been mostly noted in high-risk patients, specifically in those with left ventricular hypertrophy, left ventricular dysfunction, and postmyocardial infarction.

Beta-blockers are shown to be effective for rate control and probably for maintenance of sinus rhythm. However, the data related to their use for preventing new-onset AF is limited. The possible mechanisms of action of beta-blockers to this effect may include preventing adverse remodeling and ischemia reduced sympathetic drive or counteraction of the β-adrenergic shortening of action potential that otherwise could result in perpetuation of AF.

Data related to the other drug classes, such as calcium channel blockers and diuretics, is limited.

KEY POINTS

- There exists an increased risk of AF in the patients who have hypertension. In AF trials, the most common disorder is hypertension.
- Generally, atrial fibrillation is a progressive disease, which usually gets worsen with time ("atrial fibrillation begets atrial fibrillation"). This worsening is caused due to electrical, contractile as well as structural changes in the atria, which is called as atrial remodeling.
- Atrial fibrillation results in decreased cardiac function and enhanced risk of thromboembolism.
- There is a requirement of prevention and novel treatment regimens of AF, keeping in mind the increase in old age population, increased percentage of uncontrolled hypertension, the risk of stroke as well as the worsening of other existing comorbidities in the presence of AF.

SUGGESTED READING

1. Manolis AJ, Rosei EA EA, Coca A, et al. Hypertension and atrial fibrillation: diagnostic approach, prevention and treatment. Position paper of the Working Group' Hypertension Arrhythmias and Thrombosis' of the European Society of Hypertension. J Hypertens. 2012;30(2):239-52.

What is New in Indian Guidelines on Hypertension-IV?

- The title of "Indian Guidelines on Hypertension (IGH-IV)" will be used for the 2019 guidelines henceforth.
- The health related toxic effects of mercury are recognized world over and mercury sphygmomanometers are being replaced by aneroid and digital oscillometric sphygmomanometers.
- The change is inevitable and Indian physicians should also move towards using these devices and wean off the use of mercury sphygmomanometers.
- HBPM should be encouraged for better patient involvement and compliance. Reliable oscillometric devices should be used.
- HBPM correlates better with HMOD than the office recordings.
- Masked hypertension also needs to be diagnosed and recognized like the white coat hypertension we have been more familiar with.
- The diagnosis of hypertension will be blood pressure of ≥140/90 for office BP.
- HBPM and ABPM readings are lower than office readings. The diagnosis by HBPM and by mean daytime ABPM will be pressure of >135/85 and a 24-hour mean ABPM of >130/80.
- The latest data in India shows that presently the prevalence in urban areas is 33.8% and, in rural areas, it is 27.6% with an overall prevalence of 29.8%.
- Prevalence of hypertension is increasing in India as against some other nations since our longevity is increasing.
- The levels of control of blood pressure are very low at 20% in urban and 11% in rural population. Large public health measures need to be undertaken to improve this.
- Special features of hypertension in India have been included and discussed for the first time.
- ACEIs and ARBs are the preferred agents in young (<60 years), and CCBs and diuretics are the preferred agents in those >60 years.
- Combination therapy in single pill is encouraged for better compliance. >70% patients need combination of drugs for control of blood pressure.
- We should start with a two-drug combination, preferably in a single pill for stage 2 hypertension.
- The value of beta-blockers as first-line agents in hypertension has receded and these are now recommended as agents for use in specific indications.
- For routine patients these are no longer recommended as first line agents.
- Some combinations are preferred. ACEIs/ARBs in combination with CCBs are considered a first line combination.
- Diuretics may be used as third agent in combination.
- Treatment of hypertension even in octogenarians (>80 years) has been showed to be beneficial (newer data) and is recommended.

- After the recent SPRINT study and the HOPE III study, the threshold for starting antihypertensive therapy and the target blood pressure has been lowered as compared to the IGH-III guidelines.
- The threshold for starting antihypertensive drugs should be 140/90 in most patients.
- In patients of coronary artery disease (CAD) and heart failure (HF), antihypertensive therapy may be started beyond 130/80. Target blood pressure of <130/80 should be achieved specially in those <60 years.
- In elderly, the target can be between 130–140/80–90 and it needs to be individualized.
- Chronic kidney disease (CKD) is a common comorbidity and has been explained.
- Awareness and diagnosis of this entity will help recognize the high-risk hypertensive individuals.
- Obstructive sleep apnea (OSA) and its clinical implications have also been included.
- Patients with HFnEF derive significant benefit with good blood pressure control and target of <130/80 should be achieved just as in HFrEF.
- Statins are beneficial in hypertensive individuals with dyslipidemia and should be used based on the findings of the HOPE III study.
- Aspirin has no role as a prophylactic agent in hypertension.

Index

Page numbers followed by *b* refer to box, *f* refer to figure, *fc* refer to flowchart, and *t* refer to table.

A

Abdomen, computed tomography scan of 140
Acalculia 109
Acute coronary syndrome 55, 160, 168, 169
Acute glomerulonephritis 81, 91
  management of 91
Acute myocardial infarction 126, 168, 169
Acute organic brain syndrome 91
Adrenal adenoma 146
Adrenal carcinoma 146
Adrenal hyperplasia, primary 146
Adrenalectomy 144
Agnosia 109
Agranulocytosis 148
Albumin-creatinine ratio 88
Albumin-excretion rate 88
Albuminuria 87
  management of 89
Alcohol 27
  moderation of 32
Aldosterone antagonists 171
Aldosteronism, primary 27
Alexia 109
Ambulatory blood pressure monitoring 17, 32, 59, 94
  role of 61
American College of Cardiology 170
American Heart Association 170
Amlodipine 30, 86, 89
Amphetamine 27
Aneurysm
  intracranial 114
  treatment options for 120
Angina 157
Angiotensin-converting enzyme inhibitors 3, 12, 13, 33, 72, 76, 80, 89, 91, 131, 155, 160, 164, 165, 167, 171
Angiotensin-receptor
  antagonists 91
  blockers 3, 12, 13, 33, 72, 89, 91, 136, 156, 161, 164, 165, 169, 171
  neprilysin inhibitor 164, 165
Anomia 109
Anosognosia 109
Antecedent hypertension, prevalence of 168
Anticoagulation 112
Anticonvulsant therapy 70
Antihypertensive agent 136, 168, 173
Antihypertensive drugs 34, 74
  dialyzability of 96t
  downregulation 35
  withdrawal, benefits of 34
Antihypertensive medication 133
Antihypertensive therapy 3, 82
Antihypertensive treatment 176
  downregulation of 34
Antiplatelet agent 112
Antithrombotic treatment 112
Aorta, atypical coarctation of 66
Aortic aneurysm 32
Aortic arch syndrome 66
Aortic coarctation 27
Aortic dissection 32
Aortic pulse wave velocity 22
Aortitis syndrome 66
Aortoarteritis 65
Arrhythmias 32
Arterial stiffness 21
Arteritis 66
Atenolol 86, 89
Atherosclerosis 6
Atrial fibrillation 172, 173, 175, 176
Automated office blood pressure 28

B

Berry aneurysm 114
Beta-blockers 3, 13, 160, 165, 170
  cholesterol-lowering asymptomatic plaque study 7
  intravenous 102

Bisoprolol 165*t*
Bleeding, reoccurrence of 124
Blood flow 116
Blood pressure 30, 49, 57, 71, 83, 89, 116, 125, 135
   and hypertension, effect of cigarette smoking on 20
   arterial 94
   central 21
   control 34, 102
   diastolic 42, 59, 92, 158
   effect of lipid-lowering therapy on 6
   goal 87
   lower 133
   lowering therapy on lipid levels, effect of 7
   management 169
   measurement 58, 95
   severe pre-eclampsia besides 68
   systolic 1, 15, 22*f*, 42, 59, 67, 92, 158
Blood sugar
   fasting 57
   postprandial 57
Blood vessel disorders 116
Body mass index 15, 70
Brain natriuretic peptide 155
Brainstem 101
Breastfeeding mothers drug for 78*t*
Breath, severe shortness of 174
Breathlessness 77
Broca's aphasia 37

C

Calcium channel
   antagonists 13
   blockers 4, 28, 30, 33, 160, 166, 170
Carbimazole 148
Cardiac resynchronization therapy 164*fc*
Cardiovascular disease 2, 42, 174
Cardiovascular system 25
Carvedilol 165
Caudate nucleus 101
Central nervous system 67, 107
Cerebellum 101
Cerebral
   artery 110, 116
      anterior 109
   atherosclerosis 116
   ischemia, delayed 121
   vasoconstriction syndrome 76
   vasospasm, extent of 124

Cerebrovascular accident 55, 108
Chest pain 174
Chloride 57
Chlorthalidone 30, 86, 89
Chronic hypertension 70, 72, 77, 126
   in pregnancy 71, 72
Chronic inflammatory vasculitis 66
Chronic kidney disease 2, 26, 49, 57, 81, 86, 87, 94, 161
   classification of 86
   pulse pressure and progression of 45
Chronic obstructive pulmonary disease 18
Circle of Willis 116
Clevidipine 130
Cocaine 27
Combination therapy 4
Conn's syndrome 141-143
Conn's tumor 143
Consciousness, diminished level of 117
Coronary artery disease 7, 32, 49, 53, 157, 158
   pathogenesis of 159
Corticosteroids 31
Corticotropin-releasing hormone 145, 146
Cranial computed tomography 128
Cushing's disease 27
Cushing's syndrome 142, 144-146
   etiology of 146*b*
Cyclooxygenase-2 inhibitors 31
Cyclosporine 27, 31

D

Decongestants 27
Deep tendon reflexes, assessment of 75
Deep venous thrombosis 120
Depression 145
Dextroamphetamine 27
Diabetes mellitus 15, 26, 27, 57, 89, 93, 161
Diet pills 27
Dietary sodium restriction 32
Digital subtraction angiography 118
Dihydropyridine calcium-channel blockers 17, 91
Diuretics 12, 13, 89, 130, 171
Drug therapy goals 95
Dyslipidemia 15
Dyspnea 53, 80
   causes of 54

E

Eclampsia 70, 74, 75
  management of 74
Ectopic, adrenocorticotropic hormone
  production 146
Ectopic, corticotropin-releasing hormone
  production 146, 146b
Ectopic thyroid tissue 148b
Ejection fraction 163
Electrocardiogram 25, 38, 47, 48, 138, 157,
  162, 174
Electroencephalogram 129
Electrolyte disturbance 55
Enalapril 93, 165t
Epithelial sodium channels 143
Erythropoietin 27
Esmolol 120, 129
Evidence-based medical therapy 99
Excessive dietary salt ingestion 26

F

False resistant hypertension 141
  causes of 142b
Felodipine 166
Fenoldopam 131
Fertility 67
Fetal effects 70
Finger agnosia 109
Fisher scale 119
Furosemide 89

G

Gastrointestinal tract 10
Genetic disorders 116
Glasgow coma
  scale 98
  score 119
Glomerular filtration rate 80, 83, 87
Glomerulonephritis 92
  chronic 81, 92
Glomerulosclerosis, focal segmental 81
Glucose management 103
Graves' disease 147, 148

H

Headache 41
  episodic 138, 139
  intractable 116
  severe 77
Heart
  disease, coronary 6, 158
  failure 32, 153, 154fc, 156fc, 163, 163f
    chronic 168
    congestive 162
    symptomatic 164fc
  outcomes prevention evaluation 3
  rate 25, 57, 159, 164
Hematuria
  macroscopic 92
  microscopic 91
  presence of 90
Hemiasomatognosia 109
Hemoglobin 57
Hemorrhage
  intracranial 108
  intraventricular 105
  recurrent intracerebral 104
  retinal 117
  severity of 124
Hemostatic therapy 104
Hepatorenal syndrome 90
Home blood pressure
  measurement 28, 32
  monitoring 59
  role of 57
Hormone, adrenocorticotropic 146
Hydralazine 73, 130, 166
Hydrocephalus, acute symptomatic 122
Hydrochlorothiazide 12, 73, 141
Hyperaldosteronism 143
Hyperparathyroidism 27
Hypertension 10, 12, 15, 20f, 34, 38, 47,
  52, 55-57, 61, 68, 69, 76, 80, 81, 83, 90,
  92-95, 97, 98, 100, 104, 113, 116, 126,
  133, 137, 141, 142, 144, 147, 149, 158,
  161, 163
  and acute myocardial infarction 167
  and atrial fibrillation 172
  and concomitant risk factors 1
  and coronary artery disease 157
  and diabetes 1
  and dyslipidemia 4
  and heart failure 152, 162
  and obesity 14
  and renal disorders 80
  and wide pulse pressure 41
  arterial 131
  control of 1, 139
  cuff-inflation 63
  degree of 69
  development of 10, 11, 79
  diastolic 142

drug-resistant 15
encephalopathy 125
importance of 159
in acute hemorrhagic stroke 98
in acute ischemic stroke 107
in aortoarteritis 65
in diabetics, treatment of 2
in hyperuricemia 9
in hypothyroidism, treatment of 149
in microalbuminuria 85
in postpartum period 76
in pregnancy 65
in smokers 18, 19
interpretation of 92
intracranial 122
intradialytic 94-96
isolated ambulatory 63
isolated systolic 30-32, 33f, 34, 147
labile 62, 64
left bundle branch block in 50
leptins stimulate 14
malignant 80
management of 91
masked 63
pathogenesis of 80, 81
pregnancy-induced 116
refractory 64
resistant 14, 25, 26, 29, 62, 64
secondary 93, 138, 141
severe 75
staging of 92
symptomatic 93
syndromes 22
T wave in 55
transient 69, 77
treatment of 13, 164
types 25
uncomplicated 134
uncontrolled 26
white coat 61, 63
Hypertensive crisis 126
Hypertensive encephalopathy 91, 93, 125-127
 incidence of 125
Hypertensive retinopathy, features of 32
Hypertensive target organ damage 93
Hyperthyroidism 147, 148
 causes of 147
 iodide-induced 148
Hyperuricemia 9, 10, 12, 13
 management of 13
 role of 11

Hyponatremia 122
Hypothyroidism 145, 147, 150

I

Indian Hypertension Guidelines 2
Infections 116
Internal carotid artery 109
Interventricular septum 167
Intracerebral hemorrhage 98, 102
 score 105t
Intracranial pressure control 103
Intrauterine growth restriction, high
 incidence of 67
Invasive therapy 104

J

Jargon speech 109

K

Keith-Wagener-Barker retinopathy 127
Kidney
 injury, acute 84
 vasculature of 83

L

Labetalol 73, 102, 120, 129
Large-vessel stroke within
 anterior circulation 109
 posterior circulation 110
Left ventricular
 ejection fraction 41, 164
 hypertrophy 5, 9, 18, 26, 27, 37, 41, 47, 53, 163, 167, 169, 173
Limb leads 49
Lipitension 6, 7
Lisinopril 86, 165
Losartan 13t

M

Magnetic resonance imaging 101, 118, 140
Malaise 77
Martorell syndrome 66
Maternal hypoxia and trauma, prevention
 of 75
Mean arterial pressure 94
Meningismus 117
Metabolic syndrome 5
 components of 5
Methimazole 148
Methyldopa 72
Metoprolol 73
 succinate 165

Microalbuminuria 85
Middle aortic syndrome 66
Middle cerebral artery 115
Mineralocorticoid receptor antagonist 165
Modafinil 27
Monocyte chemoattractant protein-1 12
Moxonidine 17
Multiple endocrine neoplasia type 2 139
Muscle sympathetic nervous activity 29
Myalgia, diffuse 80
Myocardial infarction 159, 163, 167, 175

N

National Cholesterol Education Program 5
Natriuretic peptides 162
Natural licorice 27
Nausea 77
Nebivolol 165
Nelson's syndrome, features of 144
Nephritic illness 90
Nephritic syndrome 92
Nephritis, acute 90
Nephrotic syndrome 90
New onset postpartum hypertension, incidence of 76
New York Heart Association 152, 162
Nicardipine 130
Nifedipine 73
Nitrates 161, 166
Nitric oxide 20
Nitroglycerin 130, 169
Noncontrast computed tomography 118
Nonsteroidal anti-inflammatory
  agents 27
  drugs 25, 31, 80

O

Obesity 26, 34
  and hypertension 14
Obesity-related hypertension, treatment of 17
Obstructive sleep apnea 26, 27
Oral contraceptive 27
  use 145

P

P wave terminal force 54
Palpitations 139
Panaortitis 66
Peripheral artery disease 175
Petrosal vein, inferior 145

Pharmacological therapy 144
Phentolamine 131
Pheochromocytoma 27, 138-140, 142
  bilateral 140
  treatment for 139
Pituitary adenoma 146
Platelet count 57
Platelet-derived growth factor 11, 12
Polycystic ovarian disease 145
Posterior reversible encephalopathy syndrome 126
Post-myocardial infarction 167
Postpartum hypertension
  life-threatening complication of 76
  management of 77, 78*fc*
Potassium 57
Precordial leads 49
Prednisone 86
Pre-eclampsia 68, 70
  diagnosis of 69
  risk factors for 69
  treatment of 68
Pre-existing hypertension, causes of 71
Pregnancy
  and Takayasu's arteritis 67
  in aortoarteritis 65
Prehypertension 92
Primary hyperaldosteronism 142, 143
  causes of 141
Propylthiouracil 148
Prostatic hyperplasia, benign 30
Protein-creatinine ratio 88
Protein-excretion rate 88
Proteinuria 87, 90-92
  asymptomatic non-nephrotic 91
Pseudohypertension 62, 63
Pulmonary artery systolic pressure 18, 41, 152, 155
Pulse pressure 44
  and age 43
  and antihypertensive therapy 45
  and cardiovascular disease 45
  and diabetes 45
Pulseless disease 66
Putamen 101

R

Ramipril 165
Rapidly progressive glomerulonephritis 92
Reactive oxygen species 20
Red cell casts 90

Renal artery stenosis 27
Renal denervation therapy 29
Renal disease, end-stage 58
Renal failure 92
Renal parenchymal disease 27
Renin-angiotensin-aldosterone system 2, 6, 17, 94, 159, 173
　excessive activity of 81
Respiratory system 25
Rhabdomyolysis 90

S

Seizures 75, 77, 100
　management of 103
　recurrent 75
Selective cyclooxygenase-2 inhibitors 27
Sensory agraphia 109
Sinus tachycardia 138
Small bowel disease 10
Small vessel disease 110
Smoking on blood pressure
　acute effects of 20
　chronic effects of 21
Sodium 57
　and water retention 81
　nitroprusside 130
　sensitive hypertension 11
Stress management 33
Stroke 32, 58, 108, 113, 134, 159, 173
　acute 107
　　hemorrhagic 98
　　ischemic 107, 108
　and rehabilitation centers 112
　hemorrhagic 99, 106
　ischemic 108
　positive family history of 116
ST-segment elevation myocardial infarction 170
Subarachnoid hemorrhage 113, 116, 118, 124
　complication of 114
　diagnosis of 114
　management of 114
Sweating 138, 139
Sympathetic nervous system, overactivity of 81

T

Takayasu's arteritis 65, 66
　management of 67
Target blood pressure 99

Target organ diseases 49
Thalamus 101
Thiazide 2, 28
　diuretics 3
Thromboaortopathy, occlusive 66
Thrombolysis, intravenous 111
Thyroidectomy, bilateral subtotal 149
Thyroiditis
　chronic 148
　post-partum 148
　subacute 148
Thyroid-stimulating hormone
　secretion 148
Thyrotoxicosis 144, 147, 148
　causes of 148*b*
　factitia 148
Tissue plasminogen activator 20
Torsemide 89
Total leukocyte count 57
Toxic adenoma 148
Toxic multinodular goiter 148
Toxicosis, transient 148
Transient ischemic attack 108
Tumor
　intracranial 27
　metastatic 116
　trophoblastic 148

U

Unstable angina 126
Uric acid
　metabolism of 10, 11
　physiology of 11
　role of 12*f*
Urinary albumin excretion 85
　three categories of 88*t*
Urinary metanephrines 138

V

Vascular ischemia 67
Ventricular premature depolarizations 52
Ventricular septal defects 167
Visual disturbances 77
Vomiting 77, 80
von Hippel-Lindau syndrome 139

W

Weight reduction 32
Windkessel function 31
World Federation of Neurological Surgeons 118

EU GSPR Authorised Reprsentative
Logos Europe, 9 rue Nicolas Poussin
1700, La Rochelle, France
Phone: +33 (0) 6 67 93 73 78
E-mail: contact@logoseurope.eu

www.ingramcontent.com/pod-product-compliance
Ingram Content Group UK Ltd.
Pitfield, Milton Keynes, MK11 3LW, UK
UKHW050455150426

5217IPUK00025B/1693